JILL ECKERSLEY is a freelance writer with many years' experience of writing on health topics. She is a regular contributor to women's and general-interest magazines, including *Good Health*, *Bella*, *Ms London*, *Goodtimes*, *Slimming World* and other titles. *Coping with Snoring and Sleep Apnoea*, *Coping with Childhood Asthma*, *Coping with Dyspraxia* and *Coping with Childhood Allergies*, four books written by Jill for Sheldon Press, were all published in 2003–5. She lives beside the Regent's Canal in north London with two cats.

Overcoming Common Problems Series

Selected titles
A full list of titles is available from Sheldon Press,
36 Causton Street, London SW1P 4ST, and on our website at
www.sheldonpress.co.uk

Overcoming Common Problems Series

Overcoming Common Problems Series

Overcoming Common Problems

Helping Children Cope with Anxiety

Jill Eckersley

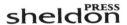

First published in Great Britain in 2006

Sheldon Press
36 Causton Street
London SW1P 4ST

British Library Cataloguing-in-Publication Data
A catalogue record for this book is available from the British Library

ISBN-13: 978–0–85969–951–8
ISBN-10: 0–85969–951–X

1 3 5 7 9 10 8 6 4 2

Typeset by Deltatype Limited, Birkenhead, Merseyside
Printed in Great Britain by
Ashford Colour Press

Contents

Acknowledgements

When I began researching this book, I had no idea that there were so many people out there willing and able to help troubled, anxious children and their parents. These include health professionals, of course, and also literally dozens of self-help groups and campaigners for a better deal for worried kids. Many of them are listed in Chapter 10. I am especially grateful to those who helped me with my research, notably Michele Elliott from Kidscape and Gavin Bayliss from Young Minds, as well as the parents who shared their experiences and expertise with me. Thank you all.

Introduction

No parent likes to think of his or her child being worried or anxious. As adults, we prefer to see childhood as a carefree time. We picture children growing up surrounded by love and security. Of course we know that, sadly, that's not true for every child, everywhere – those growing up in war zones, famine or disease victims in the developing world, and the tragic children in this country who are ill-treated or abused.

But not *our* children, surely? The ordinary, everyday kids you see playing on the street, going to school, going on holiday, in the shopping centre. Whatever could they possibly have to worry about? They don't have jobs or mortgages, they're not struggling to combine the responsibilities of work and family life. They don't *have* responsibilities, for goodness' sake.

Yet, every so often we hear something that makes all of us feel uneasy. The newspaper headlines about the young teenager who makes a suicide pact with her equally young friend. The kids who self-harm, either by cutting themselves or by experimenting with drugs or alcohol. The primary-school children who develop mysterious 'stomach aches' on school mornings. The toddlers who don't settle at playgroup and won't let Mum out of their sight.

Then there are the surveys. In January 2004, the National Society for the Prevention of Cruelty to Children (NSPCC) carried out a survey, *Someone to turn to?*, in which it spoke to 750 young people aged between 11 and 16 in England, Wales and Northern Ireland, and found that more than a third said they were 'always worried'. Exams topped the list of worries, followed by fear of street attack or mugging, parents' divorce and bullying. Later in the same year, a report from the Nuffield Foundation, *Time Trends in Adolescent Well-Being*, which tracked the incidence of mental health problems in 15- and 16-year-olds between 1974 and 1999, found that although problems of aggression and hyperactivity had remained almost the same, almost twice as many young teenagers in 1999 were suffering from emotional problems. It seemed to make little difference whether they were boys or girls, from one- or two-parent families, or from different ethnic backgrounds.

ix

So is there really something about growing up in early twenty-first-century Britain which is troubling our children? Many parents think so, including 78 per cent of those questioned by Norwich Union Healthcare in their *Growing Pains* study, who said that their children were under more pressure than they themselves had been during the growing-up years.

Anxious children mean anxious parents, but experts say it's important to get the issue into perspective. At any time, it is only a minority of children and young people who have serious anxiety problems. The Government's Mental Health Survey in 1999, which looked at children between 5 and 15, found that only 4.1 per cent of boys and 4.5 per cent of girls suffered from emotional disorders like anxiety and depression. Many children sail through their childhood and even the notorious teenage years without suffering anything more than the occasional worry. In the NSPCC survey mentioned above, almost one-fifth of children (18 per cent) said they never worried about anything!

There is a great deal parents can do to help anxious children cope, and there are many sources of help out there, too. Among them are helplines, like Childline, whose volunteers are always at the end of a phone, ready to speak to children in trouble or danger. The organization, Young Minds, has a range of helpful leaflets about emotional problems and can refer parents to other sources of help. The NSPCC exists to help youngsters in trouble and their parents. Parentline Plus, formed in 1999 by the merger of Parentline UK, the National Stepfamily Association and Parent Network, supports all parents in the difficult and sometimes challenging job of bringing up their families. And there are others, too (see Chapter 10).

Finally, there is this book! We shall be looking at the roots of anxiety in children, from toddlers' fears of monsters under the bed to teenage traumas, helping parents and carers to understand their children's fears and helping children to understand themselves. With the help of child psychologists and psychiatrists, and the experience of the organizations named above, as well as parents, we shall be discovering how to recognize anxiety in your child, and exploring what is 'normal'. Above all, we shall explain how anxious children can be helped to cope so that they grow up with the fearlessness and confidence which are every child's birthright.

1
Carefree childhood?

The idea that childhood is a carefree time, untroubled by fear or worry, is a myth. The surveys quoted in the Introduction from the NSPCC, Nuffield Foundation, Norwich Union Healthcare and others confirm what experts working with troubled children know – children *do* worry. According to the NSPCC, exams topped the list of kids' worries, followed by falling out with friends, having too much homework, the health of their families, being attacked on the street, their own health and appearance, not having enough money, and arguments with parents. Just the kind of worries you might expect children to have, in fact (and not all that different from adult worries, either). The Mental Health Foundation say that it's only relatively recently that health professionals have recognized the existence of anxiety and depression in children and young people. It used to be thought that sad or anxious children were either malingering or attention-seeking.

'I don't know why adults think that children don't worry,' says a spokesman for Young Minds, the children's mental health charity.

Many worries are centred on the family, especially in families where the parents are struggling themselves. School work, exams and bullying also make children anxious. Teenagers are often worried and self-conscious about the way they look.

Adults often don't realize how worried children can become about things they don't understand. A child whose parents split up, whose father is sent to prison or whose mother is seriously ill, may blame himself. It's completely irrational by adult standards but it does happen. A child may say in the heat of an argument that she wishes her parent would go away or die. If the parent *does* then go away, the child is sure it's her fault and she may become very anxious indeed.

At first glance, there doesn't seem to be anything very new about the range of problems that worry today's children. Think back to your

1

own childhood. Even though those days might now be coloured by a rosy glow of nostalgia, if you are honest, you will remember being worried at times as well. Children growing up in what now seem to be the happy, secure, 'cornflake-packet' (Mum, Dad, two kids) families of the 1950s, 1960s and 1970s *did* worry.

Were you never kept awake half the night worrying about a forthcoming exam? I dreamed about getting my A level results for years after I got them. Didn't it seem like the end of the world when your best friend went home to tea with another friend, when your pet hamster died, when someone called you 'Speccy' or 'Sexless', when you couldn't afford the latest fashion fad, when you were laughed at because your favourite pop star wasn't 'cool'? Being in with the in-crowd has always been desperately important to some children. Did you ever suffer agonies of shyness as the new kid on the block when your dad's job took your family to a different part of the country and you had to go to a new school and leave your friends behind? Didn't you peer anxiously at your teenage face in the bathroom mirror and agonize over the crop of spots that always seemed to appear before an important date? Or were you one of the late-developing teens who couldn't believe they would ever be lucky enough to *have* a date? If you have kept your teenage diaries, get them out and have a look at the things that worried you way back then. They may not seem important now but they did at the time.

Glasgow-based counsellor, Susan McGinnis, works with children and young people in schools. She says that the main worries affecting schoolchildren are exams, family breakdown, bullying in or out of school, very high academic expectations, illness in the family – and they are often made worse by the child's sense of powerlessness. 'The more powerless they feel, the more stress becomes a problem,' she comments.

Some young people react in a similar way to adults, with symptoms like irritability and insomnia. In others, the worry emerges as bad behaviour in someone who was previously 'good'.

Adults have more choices in these situations. If a relationship breaks down, they can leave. They can change their job or move house. Children and young people have far fewer choices. If their parents split up, their family moves or they don't get on with their

2

teachers or fellow-pupils, they feel there's nothing they can do about it.

Susan also feels that the idea of carefree childhood is a myth:

Grief and anxiety have always been with us. As adults, we tend to air-brush the unhappy times out of our own childhood. As parents, we can't bear to think of our children in so much pain. Adults don't always take responsibility for what is happening in their children's lives. After all, we have created the world our children live in. For many young people, there doesn't seem to be much to look forward to. They may come from families where the parents have always been out of work. Or perhaps the parents are putting a lot of pressure on the child to do well in exams. Some pressure is healthy, but it should never be extreme.

When there are problems, it's important for parents to be honest and communicate at the child's own level. Don't ever assume your children aren't aware of family tensions – children, even small children, notice more than we think. Children often complain that their parents don't tell them what is going on. They know something is wrong but they don't know what is going to happen. That creates anxiety and may lead children to behave badly.

Growing up has never been an easy ride, and some children find it more difficult than others. The Mental Health Foundation's booklet, *The Anxious Child*, says that there are a number of reasons why children and teenagers may become anxious. Some are personality-related. Just like adults, some children are more nervous and highly strung than others. This kind of disposition can run in families. Young Minds says that parents who worry a lot are six or seven times more likely to have anxious children. Physical illness can also make children anxious. If they suffer from a condition like asthma, they may worry about having a severe attack and becoming seriously ill, or even dying. Children with disabilities may worry about being 'different'. Family problems, school worries, and troubles with friends and out-of-school activities can also lead to anxieties and related conditions such as school refusal, social phobias and, in extreme cases, to self-harming behaviour, including anorexia and bulimia.

So is growing up in twenty-first-century Britain so much more difficult than it was twenty, thirty, fifty or even more years ago? Some experts, like Professor Frank Furedi of Kent University, author of *Paranoid Parenting* (see 'Helpful books', p. 97), point out that today's children are actually growing up safer and healthier than ever before. Professor Furedi's thesis is that what he calls 'paranoid parenting' leads youngsters to believe that the world is a threatening place. In fact, most of the terrors that make parents afraid to let their children out of their sight are way out of all proportion to the actual risk of anything happening. For example, the number of children aged between 5 and 16 who were abducted and murdered actually *fell* between 1988 and 1999 – from four children per million to three per million. The figures for fatal road accidents involving child pedestrians have also fallen quite dramatically. In 1975, a total of 434 children aged 15 and under were killed in such accidents. By 2003, the figure had gone down to 74. (For more about the dangers of over-protecting children, see Chapter 5.)

'In the past, children just didn't tell about bullying or sexual abuse, but that doesn't mean they didn't happen,' says Michele Elliott of the anti-bullying charity, Kidscape.

Some things are better than they were in the past. Race issues have improved, there are more career opportunities for girls, and fewer health worries in spite of Aids. When I was a child my friend's sister was in an iron lung after an attack of polio. I was the only child in my school whose parents were divorced.

However, set against that, Michele says that youngsters growing up today do have worries that their parents' generation did not have. 'There are more unknowns today and the world our kids are growing up in is more complicated,' she says.

Drugs, sex, complicated family arrangements, the pressure to succeed academically, the end of the 'job for life' can all affect children and teenagers. When I left university in the 1970s, I had eight job offers. That's a luxury that today's college leavers don't have. Children are under great pressure to achieve academically, even those who are not academic.

Families are less stable than they used to be and there can be particular problems for children growing up without fathers. Girls need to be aware that men are OK, otherwise the message they get is that men are not to be trusted. Boys need fathers as role models. Some parents today seem afraid to be parents and set boundaries. They fear that they won't be loved if they say 'no'. Some try to be friends to their children when what kids need is a parent! Teenagers, especially, need something to push against, something to fight. It can be very scary pushing into nothingness. Adults should not be afraid to say 'no', though many are.

Michele says that the lack of moral absolutes and a certain reluctance to tell children and young people that they have done something wrong is not doing them any favours and may increase their anxiety. 'Discipline is important,' she says.

By discipline, I don't mean hitting. I am a liberal and a supporter of the 'Children Are Unbeatable' movement. However that doesn't mean that there should be no sanctions, no punishments, no consequences of unacceptable behaviour like bullying.

In the past there were more certainties, rather than a bland no man's land of political correctness which can be unsettling for children.

Parents like to feel that they have good enough relationships with their children for the children to turn to them with any anxieties they may have, which is why statistics about worried children and teenage suicide pacts are so distressing for us. The NSPCC survey, *Someone to turn to?*, looked at 750 11–16-year-olds and found that many were, indeed, happy to confide in Mum – and, to a lesser extent, Dad. More than two-thirds, 68 per cent, said they would be more likely to share their worries with Mum, 62 per cent would turn to a friend, and 34 per cent would turn to Dad. More girls than boys confide in parents, it seems. The reasons why kids in this age group *don't* confide in their parents are illuminating, too. Many say they are afraid their parents would over-react, or would get upset and worry themselves. As many as 28 per cent are afraid of being told off and 23 per cent said their parents would make them feel stupid. What children really want, according to the same survey, is to be *listened to*, ideally by someone who has been through the same kind of problem. They also want to be believed and to know that their confidante would know how to sort things out.

2

Is your child prone to anxiety?

It's almost too obvious to need stating that children, just like adults, are all individuals, and that some are naturally more confident and extrovert than others. Many children, from tots to teens, go through 'anxious' phases and then grow out of them without any further problems. Even small children experience powerful emotions like fear and anger, and don't always understand or know how to cope with them.

There does seem to be a genetic component to many cases of anxiety in young people. If parents worry a lot, they may transmit to their children the idea that the world is a frightening place. That doesn't, of course, mean that if you have a clinging toddler or a shy teenager, it's all your fault. It's just that there is quite a lot you can do to ensure that your children grow up secure and confident, whatever their temperament.

It's normal and healthy for children to be anxious when they are facing a new experience like going to school for the first time or going into hospital. 'Performance anxiety' before exams or the school Sports Day can actually improve performance as it gets the adrenaline going. It's only when anxiety seems to have taken over your child's life, to the extent that it interferes with his usual activities and friendships, that it can be a cause for concern.

What are children afraid of?

Until they are about 2, babies' most common fears are the obvious ones – loud noises, strangers, being separated from their parents. Toddlers and young children up to the age of about 6 are often frightened of imaginary figures like ghosts and monsters. Some are afraid to sleep alone, afraid of the dark, or of specific people and things like dogs or thunderstorms. Once youngsters are more than about 7, many of their fears become more realistic. Schoolchildren and teenagers may worry about illness, injury, school performance, death and disaster. Small children can fall prey to completely

7

irrational fears too, as well as worrying about things they don't quite understand, as Sam's mother, Jane, describes:

Sam
Sam has always been quite a nervous little boy. When he was very small he would become absolutely hysterical if any fluff from our bathroom carpet got into his bath and I'd have to take him out. It didn't matter how often I explained that it was only carpet fluff, he just couldn't cope. That particular phobia died away by itself, but then he developed a fear of trains. We couldn't understand why the idea of going on a train distressed him so much, especially as he adored *Thomas the Tank Engine*. We normally travelled by car so it wasn't actually a problem until he was due to go on a trip with his nan and he became very clingy and worried. He was about 6 by then. It turned out that he was worried about what he would do if he needed the loo on the train. No one had thought to tell him that there were toilets he could use and he was terrified that he'd wet his pants.

Signs and symptoms to look out for

In toddlers – you need to take your child's temperament into account, and remember that all small children are upset when they are separated from parents or carers, and have occasional sleepless nights. However, if your toddler:

• is unable to play with other children,
• is unable to sleep alone,
• cries and seems distressed when you go into another room,

then it might be that she is excessively anxious.

Don't worry, by the way, if your child has a favourite toy or 'cuddly' from which she refuses to be parted. This can be something like a teddy or a bit of worn old blanket. This is very common behaviour and according to the Mental Health Foundation, some experts believe that children who have a comfort object like this are better able to cope with growing up than those who don't.

In school-age children – look out for those who:

- are extremely shy, timid or clinging, preferring to stay by your side, or with the teacher at school;
- have problems mixing with other children, and seem to be 'loners' who don't pitch in with the rest in the playground;
- often have problems sleeping and complain of frequent bad dreams or nightmares;
- complain of headaches or 'tummy aches' a lot;
- always seem worried and keep asking you if everything is all right.

In teenagers – remember that almost all teenagers have 'moods' at this time of physical and emotional development. Tears, sulks and locking the bedroom door while they confide in their best friend or their diary are par for the course and don't necessarily indicate a serious anxiety problem. Look out for:

- excessive shyness which leads to teenagers being unable or unwilling to mix with others;
- panic attacks and phobias;
- binge eating or excessive dieting (see Chapter 9);
- poor sleep or, alternatively, excessive sleepiness;
- destructive behaviour like excessive drinking or experimenting with drugs.

What makes children anxious?

Children who are worriers by nature may be made more so by the circumstances they find themselves in. Unlike adults, children are often powerless to change their situation, and that can produce anxiety in itself. When they are not told what's happening – or not told enough, or they don't understand what they are told, they can become even more anxious.

On the whole, children are conservative and are often frightened by change. Even small changes in routine can worry them, as can major changes like a new baby in the family, a house move, or a family crisis like illness or separation. Tension and rows in the family can have an effect on even small children and lead to irritability, whining, attention-seeking and general naughtiness. Anxious older children may revert to the behaviours expected of younger children, like bed-wetting or rebellious and confrontational behaviour.

How you can help your anxious child

The two things that anxious children most need are *security* and *confidence*, often referred to as *self-esteem*. Most troubled, anxious and even delinquent children and young people lack one or both of these vital factors in their lives. The Royal College of Psychiatrists has this to say about good parenting:

> Good parenting is about providing a warm, secure home life, helping your child to learn the rules of life – how to share, respecting others, etc., and to develop good self-esteem.
>
> Rules are an important part of everyday life. They make it possible for us to get along with one another.

Rules also help to make children feel secure, which is why consistent discipline is one invaluable way to help your child. Discipline doesn't have to mean harshness, shouting or smacking, it just means making sure that your children know what is, and isn't, acceptable behaviour. Don't make promises – or threats – that you can't keep, however exasperated you are feeling. It's especially important that both parents stick to the same rules, so that there's no wheedling Dad for treats like staying up late if Mum has already said 'no'! The same applies to Nan and the childminder. If the rule in your house is bedtime at seven, or no snacks between meals, or that children who don't eat their vegetables don't get any pudding, your children will know exactly where they are. Children who are never given clear boundaries, so that sometimes they're allowed to run riot while at others they are smacked or sent to bed early, are almost bound to become anxious. They need to know that Mum and Dad say what they mean, and mean what they say, and that good behaviour brings rewards.

Obviously, rules need to change as children grow older. Later bedtimes and more independence are privileges for older ones, but even stroppy teenagers need to know that the boundaries are there. Child psychologists all point out that praise for good behaviour works better than constant criticism and that children need to be listened to, and shown all the time that they are valued and loved.

Much of this 'positive parenting' comes naturally to caring parents, though if your child is especially clingy or anxious you might need to make an extra effort to reinforce the messages you're giving him. Plenty of hugs and cuddles, plenty of praise, plenty of attention, whether that means a walk and a game of football in the park, a bedtime story, or simply time out for him to tell you what he did at school, all help a child to know that he *matters* – which is really what self-esteem is all about.

It's very easy to damage a shy, sensitive and anxious child's self-esteem without meaning to, simply by the words you use, the way you use them, or your attitude. If you're always too busy to listen, your child gets the message that he doesn't matter or that doing the laundry or answering the phone is more important to you than he is. Children, and especially teenagers, don't feel inclined to confide in parents who laugh at them, belittle them, or don't take their worries and concerns seriously. Some families go in for a lot of teasing, which is usually good-natured but can be too much for an anxious child to cope with. If your teenage daughter is breaking her heart over some boy who has never given her a second glance, or the latest pop star, it won't help if you tell her she's silly or that there are plenty more fish in the sea.

When you have to scold or criticize your child – and no one would ever pretend that you don't have to, sometimes – there are ways of doing it that don't undermine his confidence. One tip is to use what psychologists call 'I' statements instead of 'you' state-ments. This means that instead of saying something like, 'You left your bedroom in a terrible state . . . you're so messy!', you say, 'I get really tired of tidying up after you – you know you're old enough to keep your room tidy.' It's the behaviour you are criticizing, after all, not the child. Try to find something to praise if your child has made an effort – eaten a few mouthfuls of the hated broccoli, spent half an hour struggling with his maths homework – instead of homing in straight away on what is wrong.

Children, from toddlers to teenagers, generally want their parents

11

to be pleased with and proud of them. If they're continually criticized, they will grow up feeling that they can never get it right, however hard they try. That's a recipe for less confidence and more anxiety. It can help to increase your child's self-esteem if you can help her to find something she is really good at, whether it's art, sport, singing or taking care of the family guinea-pig.

The importance of communication

Children can only feel truly secure and confident when they know what's going on in their world. Of course, parents often try to protect their children with the best possible intentions. If there is a family problem or crisis like a job loss, house move, illness or separation, children do need to be kept in the picture. Even quite small children often sense that something isn't right and become even more anxious if they're not told what is likely to happen to them. We will be looking at family crises in more depth in later chapters, but the important thing to remember is that *you* – as parents – are the best people to tell your children what is happening, and to reassure them that, if there is a problem, it isn't their fault. Children can, and do, blame themselves for anything from a sibling's illness to parents' divorce, and need constant reassurance that they are not responsible.

3
The early years

Young babies have a very limited range of fears. For example, they will cry if they hear an unexpectedly loud noise, if they are hungry or have a dirty nappy. From the age of about six months, they become more aware of the world around them and more wary of things – and people – that seem unfamiliar, and therefore scary. At the same time, babies and toddlers are becoming increasingly more independent, exploring their surroundings, but still needing to know that Mum and Dad are there for them. The most terrifying thing for a child of this age is the idea of losing his or her mother, or of Mum going away and not coming back. Hence the tears and tantrums and the refusal to be parted from Mummy for a moment, even when she's in the loo! Eventually, toddlers and pre-schoolers learn that Mummy always does come back. When they are old enough to remember that, they don't become as distressed when they are left for a time with someone else.

Creating security

Lots of love, an ordered routine, and consistent but loving discipline can all help to make small children feel secure. Not surprisingly, the absence of these can result in anxious, frightened children. That doesn't mean you are expected to be a perfect parent who never gets cross and exasperated or tired. Children love to be praised for doing well, whether that means eating up all their vegetables or putting their toys in the toybox at the end of the day. Rewards for good behaviour work better than punishments for being naughty. Calm, clear commands like 'If you put your toys away tidily, you can have a biscuit' or 'If you go to bed without making a fuss, Daddy will come up and read you a story' – which are then followed through – help to create the feeling of security, of Mum and Dad being in control, which small children need. The words 'rules' and 'discipline' can sound harsh, but knowing where the boundaries have been set helps children to feel safe. Parents need to work out what is, and what is not, acceptable behaviour, and then stick to the family rules. For instance, rules for your toddler could include:

- no scratching or biting or hitting
- no snatching toys from other children
- no interrupting older brothers' and sisters' homework
- no jumping on the furniture
- no teasing pets.

As the child gets older, rules can be re-negotiated or agreed. However much your children might complain when they aren't allowed to do something – especially when 'everyone else' is, family rules mean that children always know where they are.

Children find it easier to make sense of the world if there's some structure to their lives – a regular bedtime, preceded by a warm bath and a story, for example.

Toddlers' fears and phobias

However secure their lives, though, small children develop all kinds of fears, some of which make no sense to adults at all. It's easy to work out why your little one might be scared of dogs, if she was knocked over by a large boisterous animal when she was playing in the park. But why should your small son be terrified of going to get his hair cut, or refuse to say hello to your friendly elderly neighbour? And what can you do to calm his fears?

Psychologists say that it's perfectly normal for children to be afraid sometimes. Common childhood fears include fear of the dark, of strangers, of animals, or using the toilet. It's only if a child seems so terrified that it affects every aspect of life, or shows no signs of growing out of it however much you try to reassure him, that you may need to seek a professional's advice. Often, common-sense reassurance and practical measures can do a lot to help. Fear and excitement are often linked, as they are in many of the games parents play with young children – running and catching, hiding and calling 'Boo!' Some fears do have an obvious cause, like the over-exuberant dog, falling off a garden swing, being splashed by an especially big wave at the seaside. Children can also develop fears when they are faced with new or unfamiliar situations they don't understand, like the arrival of a new baby or a house move. Storybooks and TV programmes, even those intended for young children, can sometimes be unexpectedly frightening, or your child could have heard and misunderstood something you, her dad or one of her older brothers and sisters said. As Daniel's mother, Sue, describes:

Daniel

Daniel had always been perfectly happy to go to bed in his own room until he was about three and a half. Then he suddenly became very clingy and wouldn't let me leave him at night. I couldn't work out why, until I realized I had been closing his bedroom window at night with a comment about 'keeping the draughts out'. Poor little Dan had no idea what these awful 'draughts' were or why I was being so careful to keep them out! Once I realized, and explained to him, we had no more problems.

But you just can't tell what will scare individual children. You would think that Beatrix Potter stories would be just the thing for bedtime reading but a friend of mine's little boy used to have nightmares about Samuel Whiskers making Tom Kitten into a roly-poly pudding! When you think about it, it *is* rather horrible!

Even if you don't quite understand what has frightened your child so much, love and cuddles can help to reassure her. It doesn't help to tell her she is being silly and that there is nothing to be afraid of. Instead, you can adapt the behaviour-therapy techniques used to cope with adult phobias to help her get used to whatever it is she fears, very slowly and one step at a time. If she really can't cope, leave it for a time. For instance, don't force her to sleep in the dark if it frightens her. It can help to fit a dimmer switch in her bedroom and explain that when you turn the light out, everything is just the same – her toys, her teddy, the cupboard where her clothes are kept, and that you and Daddy are only downstairs. By all means let her have a night-light if this helps. Make sure her bedtime routine involves a gentle wind-down from the excitements of the day, with a warm bath, a cuddle and a soothing story before it's time for sleep.

Similarly, if dogs scare your child, get her used to pictures, TV programmes and storybooks about dogs before she needs to meet a real one. Even little children appreciate an explanation, that the big dog really only wants to play and be friends and won't hurt her. At the same time, encourage her not to touch or pat strange dogs until you have checked with the owner that the dog is used to children and won't snap. It's always a delicate balance between taking care to protect your child, and showing her that the world is not really such a frightening place.

You also need to acknowledge her fear, rather than dismissing it, so that she realizes that it's acceptable to be afraid of something she doesn't understand. If you do that – perhaps saying something like 'yes, I know you're scared, he *is* a big dog, isn't he?' – she learns to trust her own feelings. You might tell her that you were scared of the dark, or of big dogs, when you were small.

A fear of water can be dealt with in the same gradual way. If your tot doesn't enjoy splashing about in the bath, you can always wash him in a bowl on the bathroom floor for the time being. Let him sit in it, paddle in it, get used to it and only gradually introduce him to deeper water, perhaps by putting the bowl in the bath at first. It can be hard for adults to realize how big a bath can seem to a very small child! And it's the same with the toilet. A surprising number of children find full-size (or unfamiliar) toilets intimidating. They're afraid of falling in and disappearing down the S-bend. Slow, gentle reassurance is the way to convince your child that he is safe, that he can't fall or disappear and that you will hold him tight while he uses it. You can buy special child-size seats that fit over the regular one, if that helps.

Nightmares and night terrors

Most little children have bad dreams and nightmares sometimes. Stories, TV programmes and videos can all be pretty scary. Even if you carefully monitor what your children watch you can't ever be sure that they won't see or hear something that frightens them – it doesn't have to be a so-called 'video nasty'! Real-life situations like accidents or a squabble with a friend or sibling can also cause bad dreams. Children can often remember their dreams and will need to be soothed and comforted before they can go back to sleep. If your child has a lot of bad dreams, encourage him to talk about them or, if he's old enough, to draw a picture of the 'monster' that has scared him.

Night terrors are different. They usually occur in young children shortly after they have fallen asleep. The child starts to scream uncontrollably and looks as though he is awake, though this is not the case. He probably won't recognize you or be able to tell you anything about what has happened, he will seem confused as well as distressed, and will be difficult to comfort. The best thing to do is to sit quietly with your child for five or ten minutes until the terror passes. He is unlikely to remember the incident when he wakes up. Most children grow out of night terrors, just as those with a tendency to sleepwalk grow out of that, too. If your toddler sleepwalks, take common-sense precautions to make sure he can't hurt himself, like making sure all doors and windows are secure and you have a stairgate. It's not dangerous to wake a sleepwalking child but it's simpler to lead him gently back to bed and tuck him in.

Facing a new experience

New experiences are often frightening for small children, especially when they don't know what to expect. Now that most children attend some sort of playgroup or One o'Clock Club, going to school for the first time isn't quite the ordeal that it was in the days when children were cared for exclusively by their mums. It's a good idea to accustom your child to being cared for by other, trusted adults, anyway. That's how he learns that when you go away, you always come back.

The National Childminding Association (NCMA) (contact details on p. 90) has tips and hints for parents in their (free) publication, *Choosing the Right Childminder*. Its suggestions are useful when you are leaving your child with another carer at any time. It's a good idea to visit the childminder on a couple of occasions, and stay there with your child for perhaps half an hour, so that he gets used to the new faces and the new environment. After that you could leave him for a short time while you briefly visit the shops, saying goodbye cheerfully and telling him you'll be back soon. The next time, you could leave for a little longer, perhaps leaving your bag or gloves with him to reinforce the idea that he hasn't been abandoned for ever. The NCMA say it's very unusual for a child not to settle after a couple of weeks, though, of course, children are all individuals.

Most are soon happily distracted by toys, games, the other children, or a cuddle from the childminder.

Doctors and dentists

It's important to talk to your child and let her know what is happening, even when you're sure she's too young to understand exactly what you're telling her. If she has to go to the doctor, the clinic for a check-up or vaccinations, or the dentist, tell her just what is going to happen. Most doctors' waiting-rooms now have toys and games for children to play with. The British Dental Association recommends that you bring your children to your own regular check-ups when they are very young, so that they become familiar with the dentist and her equipment, and see her as a friend. Modern dental treatments are a world away from the miseries of the past. It's heartening to discover from a survey by the *British Dental Journal* in 2003 that eight out of ten children aren't at all afraid of going to the dentist.

Pretend games of doctors at home, with toy stethoscopes or a nurse's outfit to dress up in and give Teddy medicines and injections, will help to make any treatment your child needs seem more familiar and less frightening. There are also lots of books aimed at explaining new experiences to very young children, which you might find helpful. Look in the children's section of your local bookshop and you are sure to find examples.

Hospitals

The treatment of children in hospital has changed dramatically in the last fifty years – since the days when parents were advised not to visit because it only upset their children, who would 'soon settle' if they were left alone! Parents, nowadays, can often stay with their children and hospitals are infinitely more child-friendly places than they used to be. Play areas and playleaders have been part of paediatric care since the 1970s, and according to a spokesman for Great Ormond Street Hospital, the USA and Britain have led the way. 'Parents and children are now involved in the design of services they use,' he says. 'Visitors from other countries are often amazed at how child-friendly our hospitals are.'

The charity, Action for Sick Children (contact details on p. 85), has been campaigning for improvements in the quality of care for sick children for more than forty years. It has worked closely with parents and healthcare professionals to ensure that sick children are as well prepared as possible for the experience of seeing the doctor or going into hospital. The range of helpful booklets it produces include topics like *What to expect when your child goes into hospital* and *Helping children cope with pain*. It recommends explaining as much as possible about what is going to happen and says that if a procedure is going to hurt – an injection, for example – it's better to be honest with your child about it. If your child is admitted to hospital, he will be allocated a 'named nurse' who is responsible for looking after him and planning his care. Many hospitals also have play specialists or play leaders who are very experienced in helping parents to reassure and comfort anxious children before, during and after a hospital stay.

Your own fears

It can be especially difficult to reassure your toddler, if she is afraid of something that frightens you, too. How do you prevent your child from developing a phobia about spiders, thunder, or the dentist, if you are scared to death of those things yourself? You can, of course, avoid the issue by getting your partner to take your child to her dental appointments, but eventually you will have to face the fear yourself. How do you do that?

'Parents do pass on phobias without meaning to,' agrees Margaret Hawkins of No Panic, the support group for those with any kind of panic or anxiety disorder (contact details on p. 92).

Children often copy what their parents do. If you are really terrified of, for instance, spiders or the dentist, taking care of your child might be just the excuse you need to spur you into getting treatment for your own problem. People with phobias can be helped.

Even telling your child that, for instance, spiders can't hurt her, but that Daddy doesn't like them much so he catches them in a glass or a tea towel and puts them safely out into the garden, can often reassure you as much as your little one. The British Dental Association points out that its surveys show that children whose parents fear the dentist are one and a half times more likely to feel apprehensive about visits than the children of more confident parents. Conquering your own fear will benefit your child as well as yourself.

4

School-age children and their worries

It should be easier to identify and deal with your children's fears and worries when they reach school age because they are old enough to tell you what's worrying them. However, the evidence from surveys like the NSPCC's *Someone to turn to?* shows that many youngsters simply don't tell. Sadly, about one in seven of those questioned said they couldn't talk to their parents about their worries. Others are afraid their parents will over-react, that parents will be upset or worry themselves, or that they will be told off. 'Arguments with parents' came quite high up on the list of things kids worry about, too – as did divorce and separation, and arguments between parents. Sometimes it seems that parents and family relationships *are* the problem – so what can concerned parents do?

Listening to children

The NSPCC has produced a booklet, *Listening to Children – a guide for parents and carers*, which makes the point that children who are listened to, right from their earliest childhood, grow up both more self-confident and more likely to confide in their parents when things go wrong. Listening to a child is just another way of letting her know that she's loved, that she matters. In today's fast-paced world, when many of us are preoccupied with work, shopping, putting meals on the table, housework and a million and one other things, it's all too easy for something as simple as relaxing and having a chat to your child to be forgotten. Most parents, too, know all about the frustration of trying to talk to a child who simply isn't very forthcoming. The dialogue goes like this:

Mum: How was school today then?   *Child*: OK.
Mum: What did you do?   *Child*: Nothing.

The best way to cope with an uncommunicative child like this is to try and frame questions that can't just be answered with a 'yes' or 'no' or 'OK'– for example, 'What was the nicest thing that happened to you at school today?' or 'What did you do at playtime?'.

On the other hand, there are children, especially little ones, who chatter endlessly and ask questions all the time. Sometimes the inevitable 'Why?' will drive you crazy. Of course it's OK to tell your child that you need to finish what you're doing before you can give him your full attention. Or, if the children tend to jump on you the moment you arrive home from work, why not establish a routine where you give them a big hug and kiss and then have five minutes' 'Mum (or Dad) time' while you take off your coat, maybe get changed into a more casual outfit, put the kettle on for a cuppa and *then* have a chat to the children? Once you are ready to listen – and talk – make sure your child knows that you are interested and really want to hear what he has to say. Get down to his level if you like, or have a chat at the kitchen table with a drink and a biscuit. Five minutes' relaxing time like that can help your child to feel that he matters and that what he has to say is important to you. As he grows up, he'll get used to sharing his thoughts and feelings with you as well as telling you all about the happenings of his day. Then, if there are any worries, you should be able to pick up on them and talk them over together.

If your child seems unusually quiet or unhappy, ask her if there's anything she'd like to tell you about. Things that seem utterly trivial to adults can often loom large in the minds of children. Respect her feelings and her fears and *never*, *ever* laugh at her or tell her she's silly to feel the way she does. You can't complain that a child doesn't confide in you if you belittle her worries when she does. Talking over worries and anxieties is a habit, and if you allow your child to develop the habit when she's young, she is much more likely to continue to turn to you – at least some of the time – when she's older as well.

Is something wrong?

Sometimes you might need to work out from your child's behaviour that there is something wrong, when he is unwilling to confide in you, or insists that everything is all right. If he has been perfectly happy to go to school, for example, and then suddenly develops mysterious 'tummy aches' on Monday mornings, or seems more quiet and withdrawn than usual, or has bad dreams, or starts to revert to earlier childhood behaviour like bed-wetting, it's a sign that something is troubling him. He may even refuse to go to school altogether. You could say something like 'I know you're unhappy about school at the moment. If you tell me what the trouble is, I'll do my best to help you sort it out, whatever it is.' There's no need to jump to conclusions, it could be something less serious than bullying or a breakdown in your child's relationship with his teachers, as Marie, mother of 6-year-old Joe, describes:

Joe

I would have said Joe was a confident little boy, and when he got a part in the school Christmas play he seemed pleased at first . . . But then things started to go wrong. He said he hated school and started to wake in the night with awful nightmares. His dad and I were worried sick. We asked his class teacher at Parents' Evening and she said he seemed more subdued than usual.

It turned out that Joe was going to be a sheep in the play and had to wear a cardboard sheep mask, which he thought made him look silly. All the other sheep wore them so I don't really know why he'd got so upset, but he had. As soon as he told us he hated that 'silly sheep face', we explained the situation to his teacher and she discreetly told him he could be a shepherd instead. The result was one happy little boy!

School refusal

School refusal – sometimes known as school phobia – is the most common childhood phobia. It's not the same as truancy, though the end result can be similar in that the child misses out on necessary education. The main difference is that school avoiders tend to be anxious and fearful, and want to stay at home with parents or carers, while truants tend to be the rebellious types who would much rather be hanging out on the street or in the shopping centre with their mates.

Legally, parents are responsible for making sure their children go to school. If your child is a determined school refuser, this can be a huge problem. Even if you go with him or her to the school gates – which isn't always practically possible – you can't guarantee that your child will stay in school all day. You really need to get to the root of the problem and find out why your child – who may have been perfectly happy at school until now – has suddenly decided that she doesn't want to be there.

Sometimes the problem lies with the school, and sometimes it's more a case of the child being afraid to leave home. Some of the children who claim to feel ill on school mornings, and are obviously anxious types, settle in quite happily once they are at school and with their friends. They may be worried about a problem at home – a sick parent or sibling, arguments in the family, a new baby, a possible house move – anything that has made them feel temporarily insecure. Some children suffer for longer than others from 'separation anxiety' and don't like leaving Mum. Crying, clinging and having tantrums is perfectly normal behaviour in a 2- or 3-year-old, more worrying in an older child, especially one who has previously seemed quite happy at school. Ask yourself if anything has happened at home recently that could have led to this new anxiety.

If the problem isn't at home, it could be at school. Again, it may not be anything that an adult would consider serious, but it can still matter enormously to your child. Perhaps she hates reading aloud in class or changing for PE. Perhaps she is shy about asking permission to go to the toilet. Or, the problem could be work-related – she is struggling with part of the curriculum. She could simply be new, or not getting on well with a class teacher or another member of staff. Or there could be a problem with another child or children. She could have become a victim of bullying, in or out of the school environment.

Whatever the problem, you need to explain to your child that there is always something that can be done to help – but that no one, not even you, can help unless you know what the problem is. You'll need to be tactful. Children hate to be made to look conspicuous and the last thing a shy or bullied child needs is Mum or Dad storming up to school and laying down the law. Children need to know that their worries are being taken seriously and that not only you, but the school staff and most of the pupils are on their side.

Make sure you are sending out the right signals right from the beginning of your child's school career. He will take his cue from you and if you imply that school can be fun, he'll go in the right frame of mind. If you seem upset and tearful on his first day, he'll get the message that something's wrong here – so save those sentimental tears for later, when you're alone! If your own schoolday memories aren't particularly happy ones, it may be hard for you to convince your child that school is a good place to be. But schools have moved on, and most are happy places. Teachers want pupils to enjoy their schooldays and settle well. Children work best when they're happy, so if there is a problem, get your child's teacher on your side. If your child continues to feel anxious or refuse to go to school, you might need an education welfare officer or educational psychologist to become involved.

Bullying

Bullying has always been common among children – remember *Tom Brown's Schooldays*? It used to be regarded as just part of growing up and something children had to get used to in order to be 'toughened up' or to 'learn about real life'. Nowadays, however, the miseries of bullying are better understood and the damage it can cause is taken extremely seriously.

> No child should have to put up with being bullied in **any** circumstances.

Schools are all supposed to have anti-bullying strategies in place. If you do discover your child is worried because he is a victim of bullying, much can be done to help.

The charity, Kidscape (contact details on p. 90), has lots of booklets about tackling bullying, aimed at kids themselves, parents and schools, and lots of information about further sources of help. It says that refusing to go to school is just one possible sign that a child is being bullied. Others include:

- starting to do badly in her school work;
- often coming home with clothes or books damaged;
- coming home starving because her dinner money was stolen;

- becoming withdrawn and depressed or losing his appetite;
- having nightmares;
- having unexplained bruises, cuts or scratches;
- starting to 'lose' money or possessions like mobile phones;
- being reluctant to say what's wrong, or making excuses for things that have happened.

Bullying can take many forms; it need not necessarily be physical. It can include name-calling, refusing to include the child in games, threats and intimidation as well as punches, kicks and pushes or stealing a child's money and possessions. The organization, Childline, was set up by TV personality Esther Rantzen to offer help to all children in trouble or danger. It held a conference on bullying in 2003 in which Ms Rantzen said that bullying is the single biggest problem which youngsters call Childline about. As many as 31,000 children and young people every year call the Childline number because they are concerned about bullying. About half the children surveyed at the time said that bullying was a problem in their schools.

Bullying *always* includes deliberate hostility and aggression towards the victim, who is usually weaker and less powerful than the bully. It is *always* painful and distressing for the victim. Bullying can be:

- **physical**, involving actual violence or the threat of violence;
- **verbal**, which means calling names, persistent teasing, spreading rumours;
- **emotional**, which may mean refusing to let a child join in games, hiding books or other belongings, humiliating the child in front of others;
- **racist**, including the use of offensive language or graffiti;
- **sexual**, including unwanted touching, indecent comments, homophobic abuse;
- **electronic** – in these days of the mobile and text-messaging, bullies have an extra weapon to torment their victims.

Some children are picked on because they are 'different' but bullies don't really need an excuse. Children who have special needs or disabilities can be picked on, so can children who wear glasses, have unusual names, are shy, are seen as 'geeks', aren't good at sport, or don't seem to fit in. Persistent bullying can lead to depression, lack of confidence, poor academic achievement, isolation, even attempted suicide. It needs to be stopped, not just for the sake of the victim, but because bullies should never be allowed to get away with their behaviour.

If you discover your child is being bullied ...

Always take what your child says seriously. Don't laugh it off or make her feel it doesn't matter. Make time to talk to your child and find out what exactly has been going on. It might seem to be a minor problem if the bullying is 'only' something like name-calling or teasing, but if it's upsetting your child, then it matters. As the Kidscape literature says, bullying makes children feel vulnerable and powerless, it damages their self-esteem and can make them feel that they don't deserve anything better. It's up to parents, family and friends to convince a child that whatever may have happened at school, it is not her fault and that you are one hundred per cent behind her.

You can offer your child useful tips on coping with the bullying like:

- simply saying 'no' and walking away;
- not reacting in any way to taunts and teasing;
- responding to insults with a bland response like 'Maybe' or 'That's what you think';
- not taking precious possessions to school;
- staying with a group rather than allowing himself to be 'cornered' alone.

Meanwhile, do everything you can to encourage him and build up his self-confidence at home. This means lots of hugs and praise for things he's good at. Why not offer him opportunities to take part in out-of-school activities like Cub Scouts or St John Ambulance cadets, which will introduce him to new friends as well as teaching him new skills. Encourage him to mix and make friends with other children who share his interests. Remind him that everyone is different and good at different things. If he's being picked on by stronger, sportier children, remind him that football skills aren't everything. The local Council sports centre might offer other physical activities he could enjoy – perhaps trampolining or one of the martial arts. Teach him to say 'no' in an assertive way – politely and firmly. Self-defence classes are another possibility. Even if he never needs to use the skills he learns, he'll feel more confident.

What about the school?

If the bullying is happening in or around school, the school must be told about it. Your child may not want you to tell, probably because she's afraid it will make the bullying worse. You have to reassure her that not only her family, but the school authorities are also on her side. Research has shown that there is far less bullying in schools which have a clear anti-bullying policy and where teachers, non-teaching staff, parents and pupils take a stand against it.

Contact your child's class teacher and explain what has been happening – with detailed evidence if possible – and ask what the school's policy is on dealing with bullying. Schools have all kinds of strategies for dealing with it. Some schools have 'bully courts' where the children themselves decide how to deal with the bullies; others have mentoring or peer support schemes where older pupils are made responsible for younger ones, who then have someone to turn to if the bullying continues. 'Bully boxes', where children can put a written complaint about another child's behaviour, are another option.

Bullying is a subject that can be discussed in PSHE lessons or in 'circle time' sessions. Individual classes or whole schools can then work out the rules for acceptable and unacceptable behaviour.

All schools can obtain anti-bullying packs from the Department of Education and Skills Publications Department (contact details on p. 88). If your child's school doesn't have such a pack, or don't seem interested in tackling the problem, you can approach the Board of Governors or the Local Authority. As a last resort, there is the possibility of sending your child to a different school or educating her at home. The organization, Education Otherwise (contact details on p. 89), can send you information about how to do this. Many home-educated children were taken out of mainstream schools because of bullying, though the general feeling among education experts is that it's better to tackle the problem in school.

Other school worries

Bullying isn't the only aspect of school life which worries children. Difficulties with schoolwork, being afraid of letting parents down by not achieving high marks, falling out with friends, can all worry sensitive children. If your child has developed the habit of talking things over with you, he'll be more inclined to turn to you for help and sympathy. Again, listening to your child, taking his worries seriously even if they seem trivial to you, will reassure him that you understand. Children who feel secure and are confident that they are loved for themselves – irrespective of whether they're top of the class, super-talented at sport, art or music, or if they're accepted at the 'right' secondary school – are generally happy children.

'I was horrified when I realized how competitive parents can be,' says Christine, mother of 10-year-old James:

We live in quite a well-off area and several of our friends began sending their children to fee-paying boarding schools when they were 7 or 8. James became quite neurotic about it and kept asking me if we were going to send him away too. Luckily, in a way, I'd been sent to boarding-school myself and hated it so there was no way I was going to inflict it on my children. When it came to choosing secondary schools there was so much competition to get children into the schools highest up in the League tables, it must have rubbed off on the kids.

My husband and I want the best for James and his sister but we don't want to put that much pressure on them. Results are important, but so is peace of mind!

Children today are exposed to a huge amount of media coverage on TV and in the papers, and can be aware of what's happening in the world from a young age. Arguments have always raged among parents about how much children should be protected from life's difficulties and horrors. (For more information about keeping children safe and the dangers of over-protecting them, see Chapter 5.) There is evidence that children worry about becoming crime victims and about 'stranger danger', and it is, of course, important that they are given coping strategies. However, they also need to know that the chances of anything truly terrible happening to them, or to anyone they love, are small. Crime rates are falling, and as TV *Crimewatch* presenter, Nick Ross, always says, the kind of serious, violent crimes – especially those involving children – featured on the programme, are actually very rare. That's why they hit the headlines.

Coping with change

Life events like moving house and changing schools can also make children very anxious, especially as they usually have no choice in the matter. Children are made anxious by uncertainty. They also take their cue from the way their parents feel and behave, so if there is a new job and house move in the offing, make sure your children are kept in the picture.

Children are generally conservative creatures and don't want things to change. You may feel the same! Reassure your child that it's OK to feel sad about leaving her old home and friends, but be positive about the new friends she will make. Perhaps you can visit the new city/town/district and find out a bit more about what it's like. Point out the good things about the move – the children can have their own rooms, you'll be nearer to Gran and Grandad, the garden is big enough for you to have a dog, for example. Even if your children are still quite small, they will like to be involved with things like choosing the wallpaper for their bedrooms. Let them pack some of their treasures in a small suitcase or backpack when moving day comes, so that the new home doesn't seem too alien in the first few days.

If you have a choice, time a house-move carefully, perhaps to coincide with when your child would be changing schools anyway. If you move in the holidays, your children may be able to make friends with other local kids before term starts. Then they won't be flung into a new school where they don't know anyone. Psychologists have identified a condition called 'relocation stress' which can affect families when they move house. Expect your children to be upset, tearful and homesick for a time. Reassure them that it will pass, that you sometimes feel the same, and that eventually the new house will feel as much like home as the old one did. Old friends will be able to come and visit and there are letters, phone calls, texts and emails to enable them to keep in touch. As far as you can, keep to the same routines – bedtimes and so on – in the new house, to help establish a feeling of security.

'If you worry and get upset about moving, the children will too,' says Jean, an Army wife who has moved house 15 times during her married life.

It's an accepted part of Service life but it can sometimes be difficult for children, which is why we sent our sons to boarding school. They went to five different primary schools and we felt they needed some continuity and security after they were 11. We have always talked everything over with the boys and pointed out the advantages of living in different places, like the chance to explore somewhere new.

Changing schools

The biggest change in most children's school life comes at 11, when they leave primary and go on to secondary school. It's not just a different school, it's a different style of learning. Instead of being in one class with one teacher for all subjects, they are moving round the school and being taught by different teachers. Those 10-year-olds who were the big ones suddenly become 11-year-old little ones again. They may be in an unfamiliar part of town, with a longer journey to school, and will certainly be in a bigger school with hundreds of other children. It's no wonder many youngsters find it daunting.

Parentline Plus, the parents' support group, has information and leaflets about helping children to settle well in secondary school. Its tips are equally useful for children changing schools at any stage. It suggests:

• practising the journey to the new school a few times beforehand if you can, so that your child knows her way around;

- finding another child who lives locally and goes to the same school so that your child has a travelling companion;
- reminding your child to take care of his bus pass and providing him with emergency money and a phone card in case he loses his pass or gets lost.

Parentline Plus also recommends discussing the choice of secondary school with the child so that he feels committed to the school he goes to, whether or not it's your first choice. Many schools organize 'taster days' for new Year 7s so that they can meet the teachers before they go to the school. Make sure your child knows who to contact if he has any problems – for instance if he loses his way. Tell the school in plenty of time if your child has any kind of special needs (asthma? allergies? a special diet?). You can reassure him in the early days by letting him know that it's perfectly natural to feel nervous and strange when you first start a new school. Many of his new classmates will be feeling just as uncertain of themselves. That's better than telling him there's nothing to worry about or that he's silly to be anxious.

Above all, don't fuss – however tempted you are! Your child will take his cue from you and if you seem calm and cheerful about the changes you're all going through, he'll cope with them too. Children are easily embarrassed and hate to be made to look conspicuous. No one wants to be the boy (or girl) whose mum made a fuss on the first day of term.

5

Overprotected children – the debate

One of the trickiest dilemmas faced by parents is striking a balance between keeping children safe, and allowing them to develop confidence and coping strategies that will help them to face the world they are growing up in. In 2004, the Royal Bank of Scotland (RBOS) and NatWest launched a £3 million scheme to improve school playgrounds across the UK. An NOP survey in connection with this scheme revealed that British parents are extremely protective of their youngsters, and that for many children, the days of spending long hours 'playing out' are a thing of the past. The survey revealed some worrying statistics, for example:

- a third of British children never go outside their homes alone;
- three-quarters of parents thought that the risks of playing out are growing, compared with even five years ago;
- two-thirds of parents felt anxious when their children went beyond the front gate;
- 97 per cent of children have been warned about the dangers of playing outside.

'My daughter doesn't let my grandchildren play outdoors at all,' said one grandfather.

> When I compare it with my own childhood . . . we lived beside a main road and near a railway line *and* the Leeds & Liverpool Canal, and we all played outside from the age of 3 or 4. The big ones looked out for the little ones and I don't remember any child having an accident. I sometimes wonder how today's kids are ever going to develop any road sense.

Other surveys have revealed similar findings, with the average 8-year-old going no further than 100 yards from the front door, and the amount of outdoor space that children play in reducing by 90 per cent in a generation. Fewer than one in ten primary-school children now walk to school, compared with 80 per cent in 1971. Fear of

33

traffic, fear of crime and bullying, fear of children being abducted and murdered, fear of paedophiles, are all quoted by parents as reasons for keeping an eye on their children at all times. Surveys like the one by the Children's Play Council and the Children's Society, in 2001, indicate that these fears are filtering down to the children themselves and making some of them reluctant to play outside.

Parentline Plus, the charity which supports parents (contact details on p. 92), says that over-protective parenting is often the result of either misjudging risks, or misjudging the capabilities of the child. It runs 'Parents Together' groups and workshops where parents can discuss this and other parenting issues and share experiences with each other. It also points out that excessive worrying about children's safety can stifle them, and lead to them growing into fearful adults. Among their tips for over-anxious parents are:

- remember to keep risks in perspective – the chances of anything happening to your children are very small;
- trust your instincts and your knowledge of your own children, their friends and the adults around them;
- remember that children do often want their parents to set firm boundaries around what they can and cannot do;
- as well as talking to your children, make a point of communicating with other parents – this avoids the inevitable arguments with your youngsters about 'everyone else' being allowed to do things!;
- always make sure you know where your children are and how they can get home;
- make sure they are taught to cross roads safely;
- review the rules regularly. Safe boundaries for an 8-year-old are no longer appropriate for a young teenager.

Parental anxiety about children's safety is slowly being extended to cover other areas, too. Until very recently the teaching Trade Union, the NAS/UWT, was recommending that teachers refuse to take students on out-of-school trips for fear of litigation if there were an accident. The school which only allowed its young pupils to play conkers if supervised and wearing protective goggles hit the headlines in 2004.

'In the world of outdoor activities, there is a view that some parents do want to wrap their children in cotton-wool,' says Martin Hudson of PGL Adventure Holidays.

> We believe that children need to learn to manage risk, rather than being risk-averse, before they go out into the world. It's partly because there is a culture of blame these days, so that organizers are concerned about the possibility of legal action in the case of an accident. In fact, the health and safety record of outdoor activities is very good in spite of a few, high-profile tragedies. Our job is to ensure that children can have experiences outside their comfort level, with safety rules in place so that any risk is a managed one. Luckily there are still plenty of sensible parents out there!

Accidents are not the only things that worry parents. We are all so aware of the dangers of child sex abuse that teachers, play leaders, and everyone who works with children is warned about the possibility of the most innocent touch being misinterpreted – when, for instance, they rub sun-cream on a child, change a pair of wet pants, or try to comfort a child who has fallen in the playground. No one wants child protection policies to reach the stage where no distinction is made between a wholly non-sexual, comforting hug and an inappropriate advance. Currently, common sense still prevails, as a statement from the Pre-School Learning Alliance shows:

> Our policy is that we would always seek to comfort children that were distressed for any reason. This is very much part of the care element of early years workers' training and practice. Our belief is that if staff are adhering to best practice, there is no need for a paranoid culture to exist within early years settings.

It's not that children's safety and well-being hasn't always been regarded as important. But, in the past, accidents were regarded as an inevitable part of growing up – as was climbing trees, swimming in ponds, sliding on ice, roaming the countryside, playing in city parks and recreation grounds unsupervised by adults. No doubt, some of these activities were, and are, dangerous. Many changes have been made to children's play areas, replacing hard concrete and asphalt surfaces with wood chips and making play equipment from softer, safer materials. Today's children are more likely to be indoors. The RBOS/NatWest survey found that almost half of all children spend more than three hours a day watching TV and playing computer games, and one in ten spend more than 5 hours. If they go out they are ferried, by car, to carefully supervised activities which involve no risk.

Even more extreme measures have occasionally been advocated, like placing hidden video-cameras in the home to monitor au pairs, nannies and babysitters, or electronically tagging children and young teenagers when they're out and about. Sensible precautions in today's world – or sheer paranoia on the part of parents? Whatever your opinion, these kind of measures are hardly likely to reduce children's anxiety. Many parents questioned by the Children's Society agreed that not being able to play outside harms their children's social and emotional development. This idea is backed up by research, including a report from the Swiss government in the mid-1990s which found that 'free range' 5-year-olds developed better both physically and socially than 'battery children' of the same age. Experts are increasingly concerned about children's obesity levels and lack of fitness, both of which are likely to be affected if we really are bringing up a generation of 'couch potato' kids.

Some experts like Professor Frank Furedi, author of *Paranoid Parenting* (see p. 97), are beginning to feel that we are wrapping our children in cotton-wool and not allowing them to explore, learn, take risks and yes, sometimes get hurt in the process. He also feels that the perceived dangers in the outside world are out of proportion to the real risk. We all remember the appalling cases of James Bulger, Sarah Payne, Holly Wells and Jessica Chapman, but in spite of all the TV reports and newspaper headlines, cases of child abduction and murder by strangers have remained stable at about five or six a year for the past fifty years. What sort of message are we giving our children, if we let them grow up believing that paedophiles and murderers lurk on every street corner? How can they grow up self-assured and confident if they are led to believe that the world is a threatening and scary place?

'Allowing children to play on their own is essential for their personal development,' says Professor Furedi. 'Children thrive when they have the freedom to explore the world with their friends.' As the father of a young son himself, Professor Furedi recognizes how difficult it is to swim against a tide of parental fears, and be the only one in your street who lets their children go to the shops or the park unsupervised.

Adrian Voce of the Children's Play Council says that its surveys suggest that given the choice, children *prefer* playing outside and that parents prefer to let them, as long as circumstances and their environment permit.

Academic research on child development proves that play is an innate biological development process in children, just as it is in other species . . . Children today need space and time to learn how their bodies react to the physical world around them. They need to learn how to assess risk by climbing, running and jumping. They need to learn physical dexterity and explore the natural environment, to hide, to make dens, play hide-and-seek and mark out their territory.

Play spaces need to be interesting or children won't use them. They also need to be visible and in the centre of the community. 'Home Zones' – streets which have been re-designed so that traffic doesn't have an automatic right of way – have been a great success in other parts of Northern Europe. Parents who are reluctant to let their children play out should get in touch with their local Council and ask what is being done to create safe, but imaginative, play spaces.

How much freedom should your children be allowed?

This is the sixty-four-dollar question, especially as your children approach their teens and want to push the boundaries a little further. You know your own child best. Age isn't the only consideration when deciding where and how to 'let go'. The area you live in, the child's level of maturity, where and when she wants to go out and with whom, and traffic issues, all play their part. Before writing her book, *Keeping Safe*, Kidscape director, Michele Elliott, surveyed 4,000 parents on the subject of independence, and the general consensus was that where you live, the distances travelled, and the maturity of the child or children involved were the deciding factors. Most parents seemed to start allowing children to cross local roads at about 9 years old, and began to allow them to go shopping or to the cinema with a friend or sibling at about 12. A reasonable age to allow children to use public transport in the daytime was also agreed to be 11 or 12. Parents were especially concerned about young teenagers asking to go out at night with friends but most permitted this at 15 or 16 – though most parents admitted that they still worried until their children came in at night, whatever their age! Clearly, it's hard to generalize. A quiet country village where your children are known may *feel* safer than a city, but on the other hand, city streets are well-lit at night with plenty of late-opening shops, petrol stations and pubs where teens could go for help if they were frightened.

Curiously, the law doesn't have a great deal to say when it comes to age limits for children being left on their own. According to the Children's Legal Centre (contact details on p. 88), the NSPCC recommends that children under 12 should not be left on their own, and that children should not be left alone overnight until they are 16. The questions you need to ask yourself – and your teenager – are, would they know what to do in an emergency? Even capable teenagers need to be advised, for example, not to answer the door after dark and not to admit that they are alone if there is a telephone call. Common-sense precautions, like leaving a telephone number where you can be contacted, plus a back-up number for a friend, neighbour or grandparent, are also useful.

Babysitters

You may remember relying on babysitting for your pocket money when you were a teenager, and older children have traditionally been left in charge of younger brothers and sisters. The Children's Legal Centre points out that the responsibility is the parents' if the oldest child is under 16. The British Red Cross (contact details on p. 86) runs babysitting courses, usually through schools or youth groups. It recommends that students should be at least 14. The 15-hour course covers first aid, but also children's rights, fire safety, accident prevention, childcare and how to handle challenging situations. The Royal Society for the Prevention of Accidents (RoSPA) has a (free) leaflet called *The RoSPA Guide to Good Practice in Babysitting* (see p. 94).

Kidscape, the children's safety campaigner, recommends that if you can't get a trusted friend or family member to babysit, you should ask your sitter for references and follow them up. This applies whatever the age of the sitter. Be alert to your children's reactions to a regular babysitter. Call them at home during the evening to reassure both the children and yourself. You could even arrange a family code word which they can use to call you if they are upset or frightened.

Keeping children safe

Kidscape has an enormous amount of advice on what to tell your children about personal safety without frightening them. One of the most useful tips is to play the 'What if ... ?' game with them,

---

The Kidscape Keep Safe Code

- Hugs and kisses from people you like are **good** but should never be kept secret.
- Your body belongs to you and no one else. If anyone tries to touch you in a way which confuses or frightens you, **say 'No' and tell**.
- It's better not to talk to anyone you don't know when you're alone or just with other children. Pretend you didn't hear and keep walking if a stranger speaks to you.
- If anyone tries to harm you or touch you in a frightening way, **run away** and get help.
- **It's all right to yell if someone Is trying to hurt you.**
- If anyone frightens you or tries to touch you in a frightening way, **tell a grown-up you trust. It's not your fault. If the first person you tell doesn't believe you, keep telling till someone does.**
- No grown-up should ask you to keep a kiss, a hug or a touch secret. If anyone does, **tell a grown-up you trust**.
- Don't accept money or sweets from anyone without checking with your parents first.
- Have a code word with your parents which only you and they know. If they ever have to send someone to collect you, they can give that person the code so you know it's OK to go with them.

---

suggesting the most sensible things to do in various frightening situations – for example, if they got lost in the park or in the street or shopping centre – as well as what to do if they saw a flasher or a stranger tried to entice them into a car. Kidscape also has a simple, practical 'Keep Safe' code (see p. 39).

The Internet

The Internet, or World Wide Web, can be a wonderful resource for both children and adults. It's already established as very much a part of twenty-first-century life, enabling youngsters to research school projects, email friends in this country and abroad, play games, listen to music, join special-interest groups and make new friends. Most young Internet users never run into any problems but – as with all other forms of crime involving young people – occasional cases do hit the headlines. Internet service providers (ISPs) can't police everyone. There have been cases where children have accessed unsuitable material – violent or sexual – or been contacted by adults claiming to be young people in teen chatrooms. Email bullying or harassment can also worry youngsters. A two-year study of more than 1,500 9–19-year-olds by the London School of Economics found that 57 per cent had seen pornography – mostly 'by accident' – though few were worried by this. A third had received 'unwanted sexual or nasty comments' online or by text message. Two-thirds of the older kids, aged 12–19, had tried to hide their online activity from their parents.

To ensure that your children's Internet use is enjoyable, safe and rewarding for them you need to take the same common-sense approach as you do to any other possible risk. Above all, keep a dialogue going with your children. Don't just let them spend hours and hours in their rooms on the Net without knowing anything about what they are doing or who they're 'meeting' in cyberspace. Just as you need to know about their real-life friends and activities, you need to be aware of what is happening on the Net. Your children need to know that they should come to you if they get an email or access a website that makes them feel uncomfortable or frightened.

Talk to them about Net safety. Make computer use a family activity that you share, at least some of the time. Your kids are probably more computer-savvy than you are and will probably be only too pleased to show off their knowledge of the Net! Work out a set of family rules about Internet use. Point out that these apply to the whole family, not just the children. Just as you, as an adult, are careful with whom you share personal information on the Net, they should be careful too. Basic, common-sense rules should include:

- never giving out details of your full name, address, school or telephone number;
- never posting photos of children on public websites or news-groups;
- never giving out financial information;
- never agreeing to meet someone you have contacted via the Net without parental permission;
- never responding to (or sending!) suggestive, obscene or aggressive emails. If anything of this kind appears in your mailbox, forward it to your ISP.

Remind your children that people online may not be who they say they are, and that not everything which appears on the Net is true.

Most parenting websites can offer advice on safe use of the Internet for children and young people, including the use of special software to ensure your children don't have access to unsuitable material (see p. 96 for website details).

6

Helping children through a crisis

Worried and anxious children naturally turn to their parents, trusting that Mum and Dad can make it right. Little ones want Mum to 'kiss it better', chase the monsters from under the bed, reassure them that everything is going to be all right. Older children learn that Mum and Dad can help with their worries too, whether it's just by offering a sympathetic ear, talking school problems over with the teachers, or dealing with bullies. Children are able to feel happy and confident when they know they're loved and that 'home' is a safe and secure place.

So what happens when there is a family crisis and that settled, secure home is shaken to its foundations by a problem that Mum and Dad can't fix? Illness, bereavement, separation and divorce happen. Re-marriage and becoming part of a stepfamily are also huge and often unwelcome changes for children to cope with. Your children might find themselves having to deal with a genuinely traumatic incident like a car crash or fire. They – or you, or someone else they know – might become a victim of crime. At a time of family crisis, you will be unhappy, worried and traumatized yourself. This makes it doubly difficult to reassure your children. Naturally you want to spare them the pain if you can, but it doesn't help to tell them that everything is all right when it clearly is not.

Separation and divorce

Parents separating comes way up at the top of any list of childhood worries, not surprisingly when it's estimated that one in four British children will experience their parents' divorce before they are 16. Generally, children do not want their parents to split up. However unsatisfactory the relationship, however many arguments they have witnessed, it's the only family life they know and its familiarity is reassuring. Just as some couples are afraid to make the break and face an uncertain future, children find the idea of separation frightening.

Exactly what worries them will depend on their age and the

circumstances. Very small children might just be terribly confused. Where are they going to live? Who will look after them? Where is Daddy going, and why? Why is Mummy crying all the time? Older children have their own worries – like what their friends or the teachers at school will say. Separation and divorce are bound to make children feel frightened and insecure. After all, they reason, if Daddy has left us, what is there to stop Mummy leaving, too? Young children often feel that the break-up must be their fault in some way. Perhaps, if they hadn't been naughty, Daddy wouldn't be going . . .

Parenting experts and relationship counsellors all recommend being as honest as possible with the children when there is a relationship break-up. Naturally, the vast majority of parents want to minimize the pain their children feel. All the same, you have to face the fact that your children *will* be hurt. It's only in those – happily rare – cases when a parent is appallingly violent and abusive and the children are terrified of him – or her – that separation comes as a relief to them.

You are still parents

Whatever the circumstances of the break-up, you need to let the children know that it is *not* their fault and that *both* their parents still love them. It doesn't matter how often you tell them, it really is important to get this vital message across. Whatever the rights and wrongs of the break-up, however badly one parent or the other has behaved, however ill-used and betrayed you feel, *you are still parents* and nothing will ever change that.

It helps if you tell the children together, and that you tell them first, before anyone else does. Unless they are very small, and even small children notice more than we think, they will probably have been aware for some time that there was something wrong and been worried or frightened without really knowing why. You'll need to tailor your explanation of what is happening to your children's ages and levels of understanding. Doing this together, however difficult it is, means that the children don't have to take sides. This is important because they love you both. It may sound obvious but a person can be a perfectly good parent, however inadequate or unsatisfactory they are as a husband, wife or life partner! You could say something like 'Daddy and I haven't been very happy living together and have decided that we would both be happier if we lived in different houses'. That's honest, direct and puts the children in the picture straight away. It's also something even small children can understand.

They may be shocked, cry, fall silent or ask questions, so it helps if you have thought through what the new living arrangements will be. Even if they don't ask straight away, they will want to know what is going to happen to *them*. Where will they live, where will they sleep, who will look after them, will they still go to the same nursery or childminder, or the same school? Will their brother/sister/ the cat/the hamster come too? And what will happen to Daddy, if it's Daddy who is moving out? Will they see him, and when? You may have to repeat your answers over and over again, accompanied by lots of hugs and reassurance, before you can be sure your children understand what is going to happen.

How children react to divorce and separation

Shock, anxiety, grief, anger, aggression – all the emotions that adults experience when trying to cope with a huge unwelcome change in their circumstances – can affect children too. Little children may revert to babyhood with an increase in thumb-sucking, bed-wetting, tears and tantrums. Older children, and especially teenagers, may seem to withdraw altogether and turn to their friends, rather than to you, for support. This can be hurtful, especially at a time when you are feeling vulnerable yourself. You can't force your children to talk to you – just give them every possible opportunity to do so. Acknowledge their feelings, too. If they say they are hurt and angry, they don't want Daddy to leave, and they don't understand why you can no longer live together, you have to accept that that is how they feel. It's OK to cry and show them that you, too, are upset by what is happening. Enlist the help of family members and friends so that both you and the children have as much support as you need at this difficult time.

What helps?

Nothing will take the hurt and anxiety away completely, but there are ways of making family break-up less traumatic for the children. A research study for the Joseph Rowntree Foundation in 2001 asked

44

460 children about parental separation and changing families and found that:

- most were confused and upset and said that they had been told little about what was happening, or why;
- grandparents and friends were the children's main confidants in the weeks following separation;
- adjustment problems were more common among children who were drawn into conflict between their parents and step-parents;
- many children missed their non-resident parent and longed to see more of him or her. They wanted more weekend contact as there was less time to talk on school days;
- over half the children with two homes felt positive about their divided lives, especially those who had a say in decisions about visits and felt able to talk to their parents.

You can't tell your children too often that you are both still their parents and that you both still love them. All the recent publicity gained by organizations like Fathers4Justice has underlined the importance of children having an ongoing relationship with *both* parents after divorce. When decisions are being made about where and with whom the children live in the new circumstances, who pays for what, when and how often contact visits happen, the most vital thing to remember is that the children's welfare should always come first.

Sadly, hurt and bitter parents do use their children as weapons, without meaning to. Some fathers feel shut out of their children's lives. Some find contact visits unbearably strained and artificial, when they are used to being with their children all the time. Others resent being treated like 'wallets on legs' and being expected to pay to support children they aren't allowed to see. If Dad walks out or finds someone else and isn't supporting the children financially, or if he is unreliable about visiting, some mothers say right, that's it, and make it impossible for him to see the children at all. Some children insist that they don't want to see Dad anyway, which is often their way of letting their parents know they are unhappy and angry about what has happened.

It's understandable for hurt people to want to punish someone or seek revenge . . . but think about it. Denying children contact with the dad they love is punishing *them*, not just him. Contact visits are not really about fathers' rights, they're about *children's* rights, the right to an ongoing relationship with the parent who doesn't live with them. (Of course, this applies equally if it is the mother who has left the family home.)

No one would ever pretend it was easy for divorcing or divorced parents to act in a cooperative way over these vital issues, in order to make life less traumatic for their children. It isn't. But the bottom line is, you both want the best for your children. If you really can't agree, get in touch with an organization like National Family Mediation, Parentline Plus or Relate (contact details on pp. 91, 92, 93). Don't let your children become weapons to hurt one another or sad and anxious little hostages, pulled this way and that between warring partners. They deserve better. The breakdown of your relationship is not their fault.

New families

Many divorced parents eventually find new partners. More than two out of five of the 267,700 marriages in England and Wales in 2003 were re-marriages for one or both partners. When you have lived through an unhappy marriage and/or a traumatic divorce, finding someone else to love and support you is a special blessing. If you have children, though, it may not seem like such good news for them. Many children cherish fantasies about Mum and Dad getting back together, even if they know deep down that it's not going to happen. Re-marriage for one or both partners just underlines that.

You have chosen this new partner, your children haven't. It's asking a lot to expect them to welcome the stranger who seems to be coming between them and their mother or father. Far from loving him or her, they may decide they don't even like the person. They may do their best to sabotage the relationship. It's very, very difficult to make a second-time-around partnership work if the children are dead set against it. You have to remember that it's often anxiety and unhappiness that makes children behave badly. Especially if you re-marry quickly, or the children blame your new partner for the fact that their other parent left, it will take them time to adjust. Be patient.

What if your new partner also has a family, resident or not? How will your own children react to having to share their home – maybe even their room – with strange children, either on a full-time or part-time basis? Someone may no longer be the oldest, the only son or daughter, the baby of the family. Whatever the particular circumstances, becoming part of a stepfamily can never be easy. You can make it work, for yourself and your children. You can:

- take it slowly. Introduce the new man/woman in your life as a friend, not as a potential partner;
- not expect your children and your partner to love one another at first sight;
- be honest with your children about your plans. Don't let them find out from other people, like grandparents or perhaps their other parent;
- not use your children as spies to try and find out about your ex's love life. Children hate being asked to take sides;
- try to cooperate with your children's 'other' family about issues like bedtime and paying for treats. On the other hand, you can say 'in our house we do things differently' and your children should accept that;
- make time to talk and listen to your children and stepchildren;
- let stepchildren have some time with their own parent too;
- try to treat all the children equally even though you have to accept that you *feel* differently about your own;
- let all the children keep in touch with grandparents and other family members;
- remember that discipline is best carried out by children's birth parents, at least to begin with;
- involve all the children in family decisions and special events like the birth of a new half-sibling;
- remember that step-parents have had a bad press, but having an 'extra' parent can be a plus point for youngsters.

Illness in the family

Serious illness in the family, or the illness of a close friend, is frightening for children. Like separation and divorce, it threatens their security. Children are sensitive to atmospheres and, if they don't know what's going on, they may imagine something that is worse than the reality. However difficult it is, it's best if you keep them in the picture. As with any other family crisis, exactly what you tell the children will depend on the circumstances as well as their age and degree of maturity. Sometimes, the simplest possible explanation, like 'Daddy is ill and has to go into hospital where the doctors are going to make him better', is enough. As with separation and divorce, it's important that little children don't feel it's their fault that Daddy is sick. You'll need to explain that it's no one's fault or your child might blame himself. If it's a brother or sister who is ill, it's even more likely that your child may feel this way. All children quarrel from time to time. Imagine how terrifying it must be if, in the middle of an argument, you tell your sister that you hate her and wish she would go away – and then suddenly, hey presto, she is seriously ill in hospital.

When one of your children has a serious or even life-threatening illness, it's terribly difficult for any parent to remember that the other children need support and comfort, too. Not only because they may be worried and upset about their brother or sister, but also because their life is going on as before while all your time and attention may be taken up by the sick child. Somehow, you still need to make time to talk to them about their exams, their schoolfriends, any other worries they may have, or just the events of their day-to-day life.

Sarah Barrell, who has worked at Helen House Hospice in Oxford, has written a book called *Brothers and Sisters* (see 'Helpful books', p. 97) about helping the siblings of seriously ill or disabled children.

'In many families, there has been no normal family life for years, maybe since before their child was diagnosed,' she says.

Sometimes that means that a brother or sister's whole childhood may have been dominated by their sibling's illness. At Helen House I would see some of these children, either sitting in a corner being 'good' or desperate for attention.

In any family where someone is sick or disabled, everyone else's needs necessarily come second. Parents spend a huge amount of time, energy and patience on the child with special needs. Families can be helped by finding normality, by realizing

48

that they have the right to have their own needs met as well. It's important for parents to have access to respite care or a babysitter so they can take the other children swimming or to the cinema. Otherwise they miss so much. Life has to go on. I have even known brothers and sisters express a wish for a disability of their own, so that they could have the same amount of attention as their sick sibling.

CancerBACUP, the cancer information service (contact details on p. 87), has a range of helpful booklets including one called *What do I tell the children?*. Although it is written for parents or grandparents who have been diagnosed with cancer, a lot of the information and advice it contains would be appropriate for anyone with a serious illness. The booklet makes the point that children have a right to know about an illness which affects the family and that it's best that they are told as much of the truth as they can understand by someone they trust.

Much depends on the age of the child, but CancerBACUP say that it's important to try to keep to normal, family routines as much as possible, to help the children feel secure. Other charities and self-help groups also produce helpful literature for parents needing to explain illness to their children. The Multiple Sclerosis Society (contact details on p. 90) is a good example. They publish *My Mum's Got MS* for younger children, as well as *MS Explained for Teenagers* in conjunction with the Princess Royal Trust for Carers. This organization also has a website (contact details on p. 93) especially for young people involved in caring for sick or disabled parents. Children who are ill themselves, and their brothers and sisters, are supported by Action for Sick Children (contact details on p. 85), which has information about going into hospital and the treatments children can expect to face.

Bereavement

Just like adults, children react in different ways to losing someone they love. For very young children the concept of finality is hard to grasp and they may not understand that Daddy, or Granny, really isn't coming back. When you are grieving too it can be hard to comfort and support your children, and yet there can also be comfort in sharing grief with them.

Cruse Bereavement Care (contact details on p. 88) has books, videos and booklets both for and about bereaved children and, in some areas, specially trained counsellors who can work with them to help them through this shattering experience. Like other organizations offering advice and support during family crisis, they recommend that the adults around bereaved children should tell them the truth, again making the point that children's imaginings can often leave them feeling more frightened and anxious than the reality.

Losing a pet

For many children, their first experience of bereavement comes with the loss of a family pet. It's only fairly recently that the trauma of pet bereavement has been recognized in both adults and children. Children do grieve for their dog or cat or hamster and their sadness should never be dismissed with a casual 'it was only a hamster' or 'we'll get you another one'. Be careful if you use the expression 'put to sleep'. It's very easy for young children to associate sleep with death and become frightened to go to sleep in case they die, too. Counsellors working with bereaved children recommend using the words 'dead' and 'died' rather than euphemisms in any case. If you say that a child has 'lost' his mum, he might very well suggest going to look for her . . . or become very frightened at the idea of getting 'lost' himself. The Blue Cross animal charity runs a Pet Bereavement Support Service (contact details on p. 85) which can put you in touch with a local volunteer to help you and your children cope when you lose a much-loved pet.

What you tell your children when someone they love dies will depend on your own feelings and beliefs. You will probably need to answer your children's questions over and over again. Sometimes there are no answers, not to questions like 'Why did Daddy have to die?' 'I don't know, darling. I know you miss him a lot, just like I do,' may be all you can say at this time. Later, both you and your children may find comfort in the happy memories of the time you spent together, but in the early stages of grief a hug and shared tears may be all you can do for each other.

Children, like adults, react to bereavement in different ways, and in their own time. They may become very anxious in case they themselves die, or be afraid that other family members or friends will die too. They may be angry and aggressive and complain that it isn't fair. They may suffer from mood swings – in tears one moment, asking if they can go out and play the next – but that doesn't mean they don't care. They may have nightmares or start to behave like much younger children, perhaps clinging to you in case you disappear from their lives too, thumb-sucking or wetting the bed. Little ones may ask you over and over again where Daddy or Granny has gone and when he or she is coming back. You will need to help them understand that a dead person no longer needs a body and so it has to be buried or burned, but that this involves no pain for them.

It's hard to reassure children when your own grief is raw and painful. Don't be afraid to let them see you cry and to know that you, too, are unhappy about what has happened. Sometimes, just letting them talk, cry, and express their feelings is as much as you can do. Opinions vary as to whether children should see the body, or attend the funeral. Much depends on the child's age and his or her own wishes. Rituals can sometimes help children, just like adults, come to terms with and accept what has happened.

The charity Winston's Wish (contact details on p. 95), specializes in supporting bereaved children. It points out that around 20,000 under-18s in Britain lose a parent every year, in addition to those who lose grandparents, siblings and friends. Winston's Wish was founded in Gloucestershire in 1992 and supports bereaved children in many ways, with books and leaflets, a telephone helpline, help for schools and residential weekends where children can share experiences with others. The organization's literature covers even the most difficult circumstances of all; for example when a family member commits suicide. It also explains the grieving process and gives ideas on helping children get through this, perhaps by making a 'memory box' or book about the person who has died, releasing helium balloons with special messages on anniversaries, or talking about and remembering the lost loved one as time goes by. As with many other family crises, it can be very comforting to meet other people who have gone through the same experience – and survived.

'I realized I wasn't the only person in the world who had lost their mum and that I wasn't weird to feel the way I did,' said one young woman, whose mother died when she was 11.

Make sure everyone in your child's life – for example, the school – knows that your child has lost a loved one, so that they can make allowances for changes in behaviour. It's not unusual for children to seem obsessed with the subject of death and dying for a time, and to say that they want to die too. Most will come through this, but if your child seems to be struggling and is still talking about wanting to die months after the bereavement, ask your GP if she can be referred for special counselling or therapy.

Crime, accidents and other traumatic experiences

According to the Royal College of Psychiatrists, post-traumatic stress disorder (PTSD) can affect children as well as adults. Your child may show the symptoms of PTSD or extreme anxiety after any frightening or dangerous experience, like a car crash, house fire or burglary. Any, or all, of the symptoms of anxiety, like clinging behaviour, bad dreams, inability to concentrate, behavioural changes or physical symptoms like head and stomach aches, might be your child's way of reacting to an unpleasant or terrifying experience. Children with PTSD might suffer from flashbacks. They might develop phobias about fire, or travelling in a car, or about being left alone at night, or anything that reminds them of what happened. They will seem nervous, irritable and jumpy. It's possible for children to survive this without special help but if the problems persist, it's wise to go to your GP and ask to be referred for counselling or therapy. Counselling is often arranged for children after disasters by local Social Service departments. There are few psychiatrists in this country specializing in childhood trauma, though there are special clinics at London's Maudsley Hospital and also at Great Ormond Street.

You *can* help your child to recover. Returning to a familiar, reassuring routine and being surrounded by a loving family really does help traumatized children to rebuild their lives. Encourage your child to talk about his fears and feelings, or to draw pictures or write stories if he is old enough. If you are also upset and frightened, say so, while stressing that what happened was not the child's fault. He may worry that you will be angry with him for losing his bike or mobile phone, so it's important to stress that you are more relieved that he is safe. Children can be very protective. Your child might feel more secure after a burglary to sleep with a night-light, or with his bedroom door half-open and a light on in the hallway. Let him watch if you have new window-locks or an alarm fitted; this will help him to feel more secure. The charity Victim Support (contact details on p. 95) publishes a leaflet on *Helping Your Child Cope with Crime*. Your local branch may be able to put you in touch with a volunteer experienced in counselling families who have been victims of crime. Victim Support can also help if you and your child have to go to court as a result of what has happened. Its Witness Service gives both emotional support and practical advice and information about court procedures.

Child abuse

Discovering that your child has been sexually abused is every parent's worst nightmare. There's a feeling that child sex abuse has become more common in recent years. In reality, it's far more likely that we are just much better informed about the extent of the problem in today's much more open climate. Years ago, these things just were not spoken of.

However common, or rare, sexual assaults on children are – and the true extent of the crime will probably never be known – it isn't much help when it's *your* child who has become a victim. Child-safety charity, Kidscape, says that in three-quarters of the cases reported to the police, the abuser is known to the child. This seems like a double betrayal, as the child has been taken advantage of by someone whom he or she likes and trusts, and may even love.

Children who have been abused may exhibit all the symptoms of anxiety mentioned elsewhere, like sleeplessness, bad dreams, and behavioural changes. They may also start to behave in an inappropriately sexual way, have physical symptoms like discomfort or soreness in the genital area, or seem frightened of being left with a particular uncle or babysitter.

Finding out that your child has been abused may leave you feeling a mixture of shock, guilt at not being able to protect him or her, horror, disbelief, numbness, and hatred for the person who has dared to do this. If you want to help your child to survive, though, the most reassuring things you can do are:

- show, and say, that you are glad the child told you and assure her that she was right to do so, whatever her abuser said;
- try to remain calm. Your child has turned to you because she couldn't cope alone. She needs to know that you are in control and you can help her. This reinforces her awareness that she was right to tell you;
- believe what she says. Young children very rarely lie about sexual abuse;
- reassure her that, whatever the abuser said, it was not your child's fault that this happened. *The abuser is to blame*;
- listen to what she says but don't press her for details;
- don't try to cope alone. You may wish to involve the police, your GP and/or the Social Services. Organizations like the NSPCC, Parentline Plus and Kidscape can also offer help and support;
- remember that you, your family, and the abused child *can* survive and recover from this experience.

7

The anxious teenager

In the NSPCC survey of 2004, *Someone to turn to?*, more than a third of young teenagers said they were 'always worried'. A poll commissioned by teen magazine, *Bliss*, in early 2005, found that the vast majority of its young readers were struggling with issues like depression, worries over schoolwork and the pressure to look good. It seems clear that the early teenage years, especially, are an anxious time.

Thinking back to your own early teens may help you to understand why this should be. If you have kept any of your old teenage diaries, take a look at one of them and you will understand what your teenagers are going through. Teenagers have no sense of proportion and no idea that time heals. When you are 14, every setback seems like the end of the world. Failing an exam means that you are a total failure. A casual, unkind remark from one of the pretty, popular girls or one of the sports stars among the guys can crush your self-esteem and leave you brooding over it for weeks. A crop of spots before an important date can make you feel like a social outcast – and that's if you're one of the lucky few who actually gets a date. Many teenagers are stuck at home on a Saturday night, feeling that the rest of the world is out having fun while they turn to a tongue-tied jelly if a member of the opposite sex even looks at them.

Those racing hormones can turn a once-amenable little girl into a sulky, stroppy little madam, and the cheerful little boy you once knew into a morose stranger who communicates only in grunts. No wonder some parents feel they hardly know their children any more when adolescence strikes. It can be difficult for you – but it's also difficult for them.

Teenagers are being pulled in several directions at once. Part of them still wants your love and approval, even though it may not seem like it! Part of them wants to be independent, to learn and experiment and find out about the bewildering new adult world out there. Many parents worry that there are more choices – and more temptations – for their teenagers today than ever before. Easily available drink, drugs, a more open and less furtive attitude to sex, terrific pressure to succeed at school and college, competition for the best jobs, it's no wonder that teenagers worry. As a concerned parent, you want to help, but how can you when any well-meant advice is greeted with bored sighs and an 'Oh Mum, don't *fuss* . . .'

However, there is good news. Not all young people turn into Harry Enfield's 'Kevin the Teenager' when those hormones kick in. It might not seem like it, but most teens love and admire their parents and want their approval just as much as they did when they were younger. They're just reluctant to show it. It's not cool. Teens are extremely likely to be influenced by the way their parents behave and they are quick to spot hypocrisy – for instance, they won't welcome a lecture on the dangers of drugs from a parent who drinks and smokes. The first reaction from a teenager who gets into any sort of trouble is often 'My mum will kill me!' You *do* matter to your teenager and you *can* help them through the anxieties of these sometimes turbulent years.

One very important way to reassure anxious teenagers is to continue to *be a parent*. Experts working with young people agree that teenagers don't necessarily want their parents to be friends. They already have friends. They may grumble and complain if you refuse to let them stay out late, ride a motorbike or hold a party, but they will be reassured at the same time. That's what parents are supposed to do! Deep down, they might know perfectly well that they couldn't cope with an amorous drunk or a crowd of boisterous gatecrashers, so it's convenient to be able to tell their friends 'Sorry, Mum and Dad won't let me!' Just like younger children, teenagers need boundaries and discipline. They need to know where they are, what is acceptable behaviour and what isn't.

That doesn't mean that you can lay down the law and continue to treat your teens as if they were little children. An ultra-strict upbringing is almost bound to lead to a rebellious break-out at some stage. There's a time to say 'no' – to inappropriate and dangerous behaviour like binge-drinking or staying out all night – and a time to relax the rules, for instance if your teen is desperate for the latest fashion fad. If your teen is basically kind-hearted, sensible and hard-working, it doesn't really matter if he or she has a bright magenta top-knot, trousers that always seem to be in danger of slipping down, and four ear-rings in each pierced ear. (Though you could offer a gentle reminder that a different 'look' might be more appropriate for a job interview . . .)

Worries about schoolwork

What do teenagers worry about? Schoolwork and exams come way up at the top of the list according to the NSPCC and the *Bliss* survey, where most of the girls questioned admitted they had cried over their homework. What with SATs, GCSEs, AS and A levels, today's teenagers are tested and examined to within an inch of their lives. Some schools are academic powerhouses where anything less than a string of A* grades is seen as failure. It's natural to want to see your child fulfil her potential but no one really needs that kind of pressure. If homework and exam nerves seem to be getting the better of your teenager it could be time for *all* of you to sit back, take it easy and remind each other that results and grades aren't the only things that matter.

You can't do your teen's coursework or revision for him, but you can suggest sources of help, including the local library, the Internet and reference books. Revision aids for exam subjects are widely available. You could help to draw up a revision timetable, with lists of subjects, charts, dates and topics to be ticked off when they are completed. You can go through past exam papers, making sure that he knows what kind of answers the examiners are looking for. If a student is really struggling, you might need to make a tactful call to the school to find out where the problem lies.

Through all this, your teenager needs to know that you love him and value him, not just his A level achievements. Teenagers need time off, time away from homework and revision, time to take part in a hobby they enjoy whether that's a computer game or going out with friends. They need exercise as well; even the least sporty kid benefits from walking the dog, going for a swim or taking up a 'different' activity like fencing or martial arts. Teenage girls, in particular, are often reluctant to take part in organized sports and games in spite of their obsession with looks and body shape.

Problems at school?

Teenagers may also worry about schoolwork if they're not academic and can't keep up. If your child seems to be struggling, he or she may assume a 'don't care' attitude which can be difficult to deal with. Skimped or forgotten homework, rows with teachers and generally bad behaviour can also be symptoms of anxiety. No one really wants to be a school drop-out and most kids realize that without qualifications they face an uncertain future. The way to deal with this is to communicate – with your teen, and then with the school. Laying down the law doesn't work. It's better if you listen to your child's point of view. A levels and university aren't for everyone. Richard Branson didn't go to university and Debbie Moore, founder of the Pineapple Dance Centres, doesn't have an exam pass to her name. If your teenager has other plans, vocational training may be more appropriate. Call Learndirect (contact details on p. 90) for more information. The simple fact that you are taking your teen's views and opinions seriously will help to get some genuine communication going between you, which should reassure you both.

Crime, violence and bullying

Being attacked is a real worry for many teenagers – 69 per cent of the NSPCC survey respondents mentioned this. Sadly, it seems that young teenagers are at risk – according to a 2003 survey from Victim Support, one in four 12–16-year-olds had experience of violence, theft or assault. Fear of crime is a major issue in many communities, and not just among the young. Anti-bullying strategies are in place in secondary, as well as primary schools, so if you learn that bullying is an issue in your child's school, make sure the school knows and is taking appropriate action.

Many of the ideas already mentioned in Chapter 4 to combat bullying can be adapted for older children and teenagers. In some areas, gangs are a part of teenage life. It's important for some youngsters – often, but not exclusively, boys – to seem 'hard' and show that they 'know how to handle themselves'. For some, this can include carrying weapons, both inside and outside school. Many youngsters claim only to carry knives for self-defence, but hot-headed youths and lethal weapons don't mix and the result, all too often, is tragedy. If your children are intimidated by local gangs, it's a police matter. You might also get support from your local Council,

Neighbourhood Watch or Residents' Association, and from other local parents.

Some kids undoubtedly feel safer as part of a gang. You can't choose your teenagers' friends for them and 'tough guys' can often seem glamorous to both boys and girls. The more critical and disapproving you are, the more attractive the local tearaways will appear. In the end you have to trust your children and above all, keep talking – and listening – to them. Encourage them to bring their friends home. Not all Goths, punks, bikers, heavy-metal kids or skater-boys are as intimidating as they look. For most, being part of a gang or tribe is a phase – like being a Teddy Boy, Mod or Rocker.

Teenagers who seem nervous, 'geeky' or 'different' are sometimes picked on by gangs or bullies because they *are* different. The best way to protect anxious teenagers is to improve their self-esteem so they grow up confident and able to deal with bullies in an assertive, rather than a frightened or aggressive way. Being assertive means being able to stand up for yourself and your rights calmly and steadily. It's an extension of the strategies that are given to younger children to combat playground bullying, teasing and name-calling. Bullies want their victims to cry, get angry or upset. If you react with a shrug and a blank stare, they'll look elsewhere for victims. Kidscape, the children's safety charity, recommends the 'What if . . . ?' game, described in Chapter 5 for use with young children, but which works just as well for teenagers. Discuss possible action your teenager might take if:

- a crowd of girls started calling her names;
- someone tried to snatch her handbag or mobile phone;
- he was challenged to a fight.

Teach your teenagers the same sort of common-sense safety precautions you use yourself when they're out and about, like carrying money in a secure inner pocket rather than lying on top of their shopping bag, not using dark and lonely short-cuts home, always letting you know where they are, always having their mobile on or a phonecard so that they can call you in an emergency, not being too shy to 'run and yell' if they feel uncomfortable or frightened. The Suzy Lamplugh Trust (contact details on p. 95) has lots of information on personal safety. Your teens will be less likely to accuse you of 'fussing' if they see you taking the same sensible precautions yourself. Remind them that you don't go out without letting the rest of the family know where you are and when you're coming home, so why should they?

Self-defence or martial arts classes – for teenagers of both sexes – can also help your children to feel more confident.

Relationship worries

It's not surprising that teenagers worry about relationships. Relationships are a tricky area even for adults and we don't always get it right. Young people have to get used to a changing relationship with their parents, and there are often anxieties over friendships and their developing interest in the opposite sex as well. This is an age when young people become quite secretive, preferring to confide in their friends or their secret diaries rather than their parents. However, they still need to know you're there for them if they need you.

The days when mums or dads sat their teenagers down for a tongue-tied chat about the birds and the bees are long gone. You can take advantage of an informal occasion, perhaps over the washing-up or the ironing, or after you've watched a favourite 'soap', to ask if anything is bothering them, or to discuss an issue that came up in the TV programme. If you want your teenagers to talk to you, make time for them, and above all, take their worries seriously. Never, ever laugh at them or tell them they're too young to worry about whatever it is. Don't give them any reason to believe that you don't understand what they're going through, or they will take their worries elsewhere.

Peer pressure

Friends can be a great source of support for teenagers – and for girls especially – but they can also be a source of misery and rivalry. Many youngsters like to be part of the crowd and most schools have their 'in crowds' who can make life pretty miserable for those who are less clever, less sporty, less fashionable, less cool. Remind your teenager that everyone is different, that everyone has individual talents and that you don't have to do everything your friends do, or everything that's currently fashionable. Peer pressure can be insidious, so remind your teens that only sheep always follow the crowd! It's easy to criticize young people for the mistakes they make and the daft things they do; equally easy to forget to praise them for the things they get right. That doesn't just mean important things like passing exams; it can also include little things like remembering to ring Gran on her birthday. They may pretend not to care, but teenagers are sensitive and parents need to be tactful. It's so much more positive to tell your son or daughter 'You look nice tonight, love,' than it is to raise your eyebrows and say 'You're not going out looking like that, are you?' Everyone, even teenagers, responds to praise. Young people who are hugged and praised and congratulated grow up with a solid sense of self-worth which gives them the confidence to resist peer pressure and to shrug off criticism and teasing from so-called 'friends'. Some teen friendships – in both sexes – last for ever; other young friends grow apart as they develop and their interests change. If your son or daughter seems to be left out of a group of friends, you could gently encourage him or her to take up new interests and team up with new friends with whom they may now have more in common.

Someone to talk to

Perhaps you're concerned that your teens choose to confide in their friends much more than they do in you. This is only natural, and part of growing up. However close you and your children are, it's unlikely they will want to tell you everything. You need to make sure your teenagers have access to sensible and realistic advice on vital topics like sex and relationships, drink and drugs. The same old myths tend to get passed down from generation to generation of teenagers! It's great if you have an open dialogue with your children on these and other tricky subjects. Again, TV programmes and news stories can be a good starting point for a discussion – and that means a discussion, with you spending just as much time listening to the kids' point of view as telling them what you think.

Ignorance isn't bliss

Young people worry far more if they don't have information on tricky subjects like sex and drugs. They may be afraid to ask anyone's advice in case they seem ignorant or ill-informed, which is where sources of information like magazines, books and leaflets come in. In spite of all the criticism aimed at teen magazines because of their generally upfront attitude to sexual issues, most offer sound, sensible and realistic advice to their young readers. They answer the questions teens really want to know about. Organizations like the Brook Advisory Centres and FPA (formerly known as the Family Planning Association) (contact details on pp. 87, 89) have a large range of helpful literature including cartoon booklets covering subjects like painful periods, pubic hair, penis size, wet dreams, worries about being gay, and anything a teenager might be concerned about.

It's the same with drink and drugs. If you and your teenagers are armed with the facts about the dangers of, for instance, binge-drinking, and the use of illegal drugs, they will be better able to resist peer pressure to join in. You will also feel reassured. Once again, it's no use laying down the law, or implying that everyone who takes drugs will end up dead. Your teenagers will have heard all the arguments from drug-using friends about cannabis being safer than alcohol and dance drugs like Ecstasy being harmless. As for going out drinking, well, everyone does it, don't they? You could remind them in a matter-of-fact way that:

- drunks are far less safe on the streets than people with their wits about them;
- girls who drink heavily are more likely to make stupid choices – going off with boys they hardly know, getting into dodgy minicabs;
- vomiting in the street or wetting yourself doesn't make you look cool;
- there's no quality control on illegal drugs – you may not know what you're buying, or what effect it will have;
- mixing different drugs and alcohol is especially dangerous;
- drugs affect users in different ways depending on how much is taken, how strong the dose is, whether you are used to a particular drug. You can't know what will happen to you this time . . . or next time;
- as with alcohol, people under the influence of drugs make bad decisions about things like driving and sex.

Teenagers can find out more about alcohol and drugs from 'Frank', the national drugs helpline (contact details on p. 89). As well as giving information and advice, it can refer callers to local sources of help. Solvent abuse or 'sniffing glue' can also be a temptation for some young teenagers. According to Home Office statistics, solvent abuse killed three times more under-20s than any illegal drug over 10 years. Call Re-Solv (contact details on p. 93) for more information about this.

Looking good

A worrying 94 per cent of the teenagers in the 2005 *Bliss* magazine survey said they felt there was too much pressure to look good. Most teenagers – boys as well as girls – are concerned about their appearance, hence all those hours spent monopolizing the bathroom. Again, all a concerned parent can do is bolster a teenager's self-esteem. He or she needs to know that being a good person doesn't depend on looking like the latest pop star or supermodel.

On the other hand, making the most of yourself is part of self-respect, at any age. This is another area where parents are unconscious role models. If Mum and Dad take care of their appearance without being obsessed with the subject, it's more likely that kids will, too. There may be media pressure to look good, but there are also plenty of easy ways to do it. A healthy diet, plenty of sleep and exercise will make the most of anyone's looks. If you can't persuade your kids to avoid smoking and drinking on health grounds, remind them that snogging a smoker is like kissing an ashtray and that no one fancies a guy or girl who reeks of booze! If your teenager is troubled with acne, your GP should be able to help. Not everyone can look perfect but everyone can have clean shiny hair and well cared-for skin, and be particular about personal hygiene. Clothes can be washed and pressed (and they should be taking care of their laundry, not you!). Shoes can be well polished. Nor is it necessary to spend a fortune on clothes. The most stylish teenagers are those who choose the styles which suit them and create their own look by hunting out bargains in charity shops and markets.

8

Helping teenagers through a crisis

Teenagers will be just as frightened and anxious at a time of family crisis as their younger brothers and sisters, though they may show it in different ways. Even though the teenage years are a time when kids are learning to be independent and break away from their families, it's still very important to them to know that their family is there – and even to have something to rebel against! So it can be very unsettling for them if their security is threatened in this way.

Separation and divorce

Research studies show that teenagers often react differently to their parents' separation from younger children. For one thing, they are much less likely to imagine that the split is their fault. At this age, they are able to understand that the breakdown of a marriage is about their parents, not about them. However, they can still feel hurt, angry and betrayed. Teenagers can also be surprisingly censorious if they feel that one or both of their parents have behaved badly, for instance by having an affair, and may 'punish' the parent by refusing to see or speak to him or her for a time. Teens whose parents are going through a separation or divorce are quite likely to distance themselves from the whole thing, by spending more time away from home or with their friends. It's their way of withdrawing from the pain.

Just as it's important to make sure young children know what's going on when you are working out the practical details of life in a post-separation, one-parent household, it's important to keep teenagers in the picture. Where possible, let them join in the decision-making. It's always tempting, if you feel hurt and aggrieved by the way your ex has behaved or is behaving, to get your children on your side, but this is *always* counter-productive. Your ex is, and always will be, your child's other parent, someone the child loves and wants to go on loving. With their family breaking up around them, your teenagers have enough worries and anxieties. What will their friends say? Where are they going to live? Will they have to change schools? Absolutely the last thing they need is additional worry about being a go-between for warring parents, or fear that spending time with their absent father is going to upset their mother.

Here are some comments from teenagers whose parents are divorced, to give an idea of how hurt they can be:

- 'Mum went on and on and on about how awful Dad was and how living with him had ruined her life. In the end I just tuned her out and told myself it wasn't my problem. I loved my dad, and knew that Mum could be pretty difficult to live with too.'
- 'My brothers and I refused to see Dad when he left Mum for another woman. That was five years ago. I wouldn't mind making contact now but I don't know how.'
- 'It scared me when people told me I'd have to be the man of the house now that Dad had gone.'
- 'My dad is punishing my mum by not letting her see us, but he's punishing us too!'
- 'We would wait and wait, but Dad never came. He never even bothered to pick up the phone. In the end we just gave up on him.'

As always at a time of crisis, you really need to keep the communication going, not an easy task where adolescents are concerned. You can't make them talk to you, but you can encourage them to open up by telling them how you're feeling – angry, sad, worried about what the future holds, and asking them if they feel the same. It's sometimes tempting, when you are feeling hurt and vulnerable yourself, to lean on your teenage children too much. They may be sympathetic but they can't be responsible for soothing the pain you feel. Being expected to support you could leave them feeling even more anxious. You have to accept that they may very well prefer to talk things over with their friends, a sympathetic teacher at school or another relative like an aunt, grandparent or older brother or sister. The NCH charity (contact details on p. 92) has a website to support and inform young people whose parents are splitting up.

Their world is changing, and not for the better. It's important for them to be able to hang on to friendships and relationships that are still the same, to keep doing at least some of the same things with the same people, to stick with as many of their usual routines – football on Fridays, youth club or Guides at the weekend – as possible. Do tell your child's school that you are divorcing, so that the teachers can look out for, and make allowances for, any behavioural changes or drops in concentration. There may be a school counsellor your teenager can confide in.

Access visits are also very different for teenagers than for younger children. This is an age when kids like to spend their free time hanging out with their friends rather than their parents. A flexible access arrangement may work much better with teenagers than a fixed 'Dad's day'. If it's at all possible for them to stay in their old home (or at least in the same area), go to the same school and see the same friends, and not have to travel too far to see their absent parent, this can make post-divorce life a whole lot less fraught for teens. Calling in informally for a quick coffee with Dad may suit many teens better than being expected to spend the whole of every other Sunday with him.

Step-families

Just like younger children, most teenagers will face the prospect of a stepmother or -father with very mixed feelings. Almost half of the teenagers questioned in the 2005 *Bliss* magazine survey said they didn't like their step-parent. They may blame the 'step' for the break-up of their parents' marriage. Teenagers often see things very much in black-and-white ('If he/she hadn't come along Mum and Dad would still be together!') when the reality is likely to be quite different.

Whether or not the step-parent had anything to do with the divorce, the idea that their mum or dad is in love with someone else causes all sorts of problems for many teens. It underlines the fact that their parents' marriage is really over. It means that their parent is – shock, horror – *having sex with someone* – which is something many teens find hard to come to terms with. Jealousy plays a part too. Perhaps you were all coping quite well with being a single-parent family, and now here is this stranger intruding on your relationship. Will you and your teenager still be able to do things together – shopping, football, visiting Gran, walking the dog, or will this other person always be there too? There can be straightforward personality clashes. Just because you love your new partner, it doesn't mean your teenager will.

Everything becomes several times more complex and worrying if your partner also has children. They may spend odd weekends and holidays with you, or they may move in permanently. Or, you may decide to move to your new partner's home, with or without his or her children in permanent residence. All these decisions have implications for your teenagers and you shouldn't be surprised if they react with anger and dismay.

Lucy, aged 15
Mike tried to act like a father to my sister and me, but I loved my own dad, and I really gave Mike a hard time at first. He hadn't been married before and I never thought what it must have been like for him, having Bonnie and me land on him after we'd lived with our dad and stepmother. It was awful to begin with, but we get on better now. I've stopped blaming everything on Mike and I know I'm not the only person in the world with divorced parents. Mum sat Bonnie and me down and explained that she wasn't *just* our mum, she was entitled to a bit of happiness like everyone else. We've got a little half-brother now, as well.

Organizations like Parentline Plus (contact details on p. 92) can offer advice on step-parenting teenagers as well as younger children. Sex can be an issue, and not just because teenagers can be notoriously prudish about the fact that their parents have a sex life! Stepfamilies with opposite-sex teenagers have to allow for the possibility of sexual attraction between step-siblings. You'll have to create new rules about privacy, locking bathroom or bedroom doors, wandering around the house in underwear – all things which can make body-conscious teens feel pretty uncomfortable.

Illness and bereavement

Many of the organizations offering help and advice to children and adults faced with serious illness or bereavement have recognized that teenagers in these situations often have their own special needs. Action for Sick Children (contact details on p. 85) has a booklet for teenagers who have to go into hospital. Cruse Bereavement Care (contact details on p. 88) has an *After Someone Dies* leaflet especially for teens, plus a dedicated young person's helpline and website where youngsters can share their feelings with others who are going through the same thing. Winston's Wish (contact details on p. 95) can support teenagers too, and its weekend workshops for bereaved kids cater for anyone up to the age of 18. Help is also available from cancer charities and, for those caring for a sick parent or other relative, there are young carers' groups (contact details on p. 93). Teenagers need never feel they are alone with their worries. As a parent you need to let them know you're there for them if they want to talk. Don't be hurt if they prefer to confide in a friend, a sympathetic stranger on a helpline, or just pour out their worries to their diary or in paintings, music or poems.

When teens get into trouble . . .

. . . one of their first worries is likely to be telling their parents. Even the most cocky, streetwise and cool teens can turn into frightened children when things really go wrong; for example, if they become involved in crime, or are faced with an unwanted pregnancy. The most difficult thing for parents in these circumstances is to support and reassure their child, while still insisting that he accepts the responsibility for what he has done. It's a hard lesson for any teen to learn, but sometimes, Mum and Dad just can't make it right. You can help, but you can't take the problem away.

Being told by the police that your son – or daughter – has been taken into custody is an alarming moment for any parent. You may have suspected that you had a young tearaway in the family, or you may have had no idea what was going on. If this is a 'first offence', your reaction may well be anger, panic, or the feeling that there has to be some mistake.

'The most useful thing a parent in this situation can do is *keep calm* and *listen*,' says Chris Stanley, head of Youth Crime at Nacro, the crime reduction charity.

Parents do not always know what has been going on, and it can be unhelpful to wade in to what is already an emotionally charged situation, either blaming your child or insisting that he/she couldn't possibly be involved.

Don't jump to conclusions. Don't condemn your child out of

68

hand or assume that he or she is innocent. Your child has the right to legal representation and the police should telephone the on-call solicitor, whose services are free. Young people should only be questioned by the police in the presence of an 'appropriate adult'. This is a volunteer who has been specially trained by the local Youth Offending Team. A parent can act as an appropriate adult but it is often useful to have someone there who is independent and objective. Parents sometimes advise their child to plead guilty just so they can get away from the police station but this is not always the wisest course of action.

If your child is charged with an offence and goes to court, a 'pre-sentence report' may be called for, especially if the offence is a serious one. The Youth Offending Team may visit your home or ask you to bring your child to their office to talk through the issues and find out where the problems started.

Youth Offending Teams also do considerable preventative work with young people thought to be 'at risk' of getting involved in crime. Such children may play truant from school and, if local resources permit, can obtain help from the Social Services who may offer family support. There are also Youth Inclusion Programmes and holiday schemes run by local Councils and the police aimed at keeping youngsters out of trouble.

If you are concerned about your teenager running wild, bunking-off school, mixing with 'the wrong crowd' and being generally out of control, it's obviously best to ask for help sooner rather than later. Parentline Plus (contact details on p. 92) can often refer you to suitable sources of help, including parents' groups, workshops and courses. Another organization, Positive Parenting, runs courses for parents all over the country, including a six-session course called 'Time Out for Teenagers'. The accompanying booklet can be purchased even if you are not taking part in a course (contact details on p. 93).

Pregnancy

More than 42,000 girls aged under 18 in England and Wales became pregnant in 2003. It's a fair bet that most of those pregnancies were unplanned. Even assuming there are a handful of married or settled teens who want to start families at that age, that still leaves thousands of girls facing the huge responsibility of motherhood when they are little more than children themselves. It's important, also, to remember what is often forgotten, that *boys* are also involved. For every teenage mum, there's a young dad. In an ideal world, boys and young men would be trained to see unwanted pregnancy as exactly 50 per cent their problem. Even in the twenty-first century, however, many lads still turn their backs, and even those who want to help often don't have a clue what to do. Besides, the girl might genuinely not want anything more to do with them, especially if the pregnancy was the result of a drunken fumble at a party. The question of whether young fathers have any rights at all in that sort of situation is only just beginning to be asked. As the law stands currently, your son doesn't even have the right to be told that he has made his girlfriend pregnant, or to be involved in any decision she makes about continuing with the pregnancy.

It still takes courage for a teenager to confess to her parents that she's pregnant. By the time she tells you, she will probably have been through days, even weeks and perhaps months, of uncertainty, fear, disbelief and anxiety. It may be a relief to tell, but she will still be worried about how you will react.

So how *do* you react? It's natural to feel anger, disappointment, shock and a thousand other emotions, but try to stay calm. What's done is done. The decisions your daughter makes now will affect you all for the rest of your lives – and they are *her* decisions. You can help and support, advise and guide, but you can't make the decisions for her. Ever since 1985, it has been the law that young people – even those under 16 – have a right to confidentiality and also the right to make their own decisions about medical treatment, including contraception and abortion. Doctors and counsellors, such as those at the Brook Advisory Centres (contact details on p. 87), will normally advise girls to involve their parents, but will not tell parents if the girl insists she doesn't want them to know. According to the law, a young person can consent to any treatment providing she has 'sufficient maturity and judgement to be able fully to understand what is proposed'. There's a lot to think about and discuss. This is a time to step back, and look at all the options before any final decision is made.

• She could have an abortion. Especially if she is very young, this could seem like a solution to the problem – and it may well prove to be the case – but it's not the only option and it has to be your daughter's choice. More than half of all pregnancies in under-16s end in abortion.

- She could have the baby and keep it. Many young girls plan to do this, often with an over-romantic idea of what is involved and no idea of the practical or financial implications of her choice.
- She could have the baby adopted. Very few healthy babies are given up for adoption these days. For every one which becomes available, there are about six couples waiting to adopt.
- She could have the baby and hand it over to you to bring up – something many Grans do to enable their daughters to continue with their education. Are you prepared to go back to nappies and sleepless nights? Is this solution allowing your daughter to take responsibility for her actions?
- How will any of these options affect the wider family – your husband, any brothers and sisters, and last, but not least, the baby's father and his family?

Sexual abuse

Sexual abuse happens to teenagers as well as younger children. The NSPCC defines abuse as 'when something sexual is going on and one person:

- doesn't like it
- doesn't want it
- didn't choose to have it happen
- can't stop it.'

The whole issue of abuse can be especially worrying and confusing for teenagers who are just coming to terms with their own sexuality and may not be too sure what they *do* want, what they like, and what is and isn't OK. Is it abusive for a crowd of guys to pass a porn magazine around a mixed classroom? Is a young man of 18 who has sex with his 15-year-old girlfriend a child abuser? Legally, anyone who has sex with a young person under 16 is breaking the law.

Many youngsters are abused, either physically or sexually, by kids their own age. In a survey of 2,000 teenage girls run by *Sugar* magazine and the NSPCC in early 2005, a worrying 43 per cent of girls thought it acceptable for a boy to hit his girlfriend in particular circumstances; for example, if she had cheated on him, screamed at him or worn outrageous clothes. A tiny percentage even said they 'understood' why a boy might force his girlfriend to have sex.

There's nothing magical about the 'age of consent'. If your 17-year-old daughter (or son) is being coerced into some kind of sexual activity she or he is unhappy about, then they are in an abusive relationship.

Whatever your child's age, if she plucks up the courage to tell you she is being abused, she needs to be *believed* and *reassured* that she was right to tell you and that what has happened is not her fault, whatever her abuser has told her.

Everyone – male or female, young or older – has the right to say 'NO' to unwanted sexual activity.

You can get help from the Social Services, your GP, the police, or specialist organizations like Kidscape or the NSPCC (contact details on pp. 90, 92). Make sure your teenager knows that you are there for him if he wants to talk about what has happened. He might also find it helpful to write down his feelings or draw or paint, or to be referred for specialist counselling or therapy. Reassure him that he can recover from this horrible experience and that he won't always feel the way he does right now.

9

More than teenage angst?

So far, we have established that children and teenagers do get anxious, and that they do worry about things that seem to be going wrong in their lives and in the world around them. According to Samaritans, the emotional support charity (contact details on p. 94), one of the main differences between teenage and adult anxieties is that young people are less likely to feel – or to be – in control of their lives and what is happening to them. Often there are practical steps parents can take to help troubled teenagers. You can enlist the school's support in dealing with bullies or examination nerves. You can help your children through family change and support them in times of trauma. What happens, though, if in spite of all your best efforts, your child still seems to find it impossible to cope with living? At what point do you ask for help? How can you tell the difference between a 'typical' moody teenager and a desperately troubled young person at risk of serious mental distress?

'There is a point when parents should ask for help, but it is an arbitrary line,' says Gavin Bayliss of Young Minds, the young people's mental health charity. 'It's rather like the question of when you intervene if your child is putting on weight – do you step in when it's a minor problem or wait till he has several stones to lose?'

Gavin Bayliss recommends that parents call the Young Minds Parents Information Service (contact details on p. 96) for help:

> Our advisers will listen to the problem and either refer the parent to someone, ideally someone local, who can help, or reassure them by saying that that's what 14-year-olds are like! You might compare your child's behaviour with the behaviour of others the same age, or ask his teachers at school if you are concerned. If your child always seems anxious, it's important to figure out with him what the problem could be. Parents can also download leaflets about mental health problems in young people from our website.

Young Minds reports that of the approximately one in ten youngsters with mental health problems, about 4 per cent have anxiety, obsessive–compulsive disorders (when they have rituals like obsessive hand-washing or counting, without which they become very distressed), or panic attacks. The others tend to have problems like attention deficit hyperactivity disorder (ADHD) or conduct disorders. These are the children who find it hard to sit still and concentrate, are always 'on the go', are often confrontational and argumentative, get into a lot of fights and are generally acknowledged as 'difficult'. Many of these youngsters come into conflict with authority and are excluded from school. Anxious children, on the other hand, being less confrontational, are more easily overlooked. Young Minds says that there may be cause for concern about youngsters who:

- are extremely moody and irritable – bearing in mind that most teens have occasional bad moods;
- give up their old interests and don't seem to find any new ones;
- lose interest in schoolwork, find it hard to concentrate, and generally do badly at school;
- become withdrawn and lose touch with their friends (child psychologists say it's much healthier for kids to have friends you disapprove of than no friends at all);
- don't look after themselves and neglect their appearance;
- eat very little or eat far too much;
- are extremely self-critical;
- sleep badly or sleep far too much.

Obtaining a diagnosis

Those treating troubled and distressed children are often reluctant to pin a label on them even though parents may be eager to obtain a diagnosis. Teenagers are sometimes diagnosed with schizophrenia or bi-polar disorder, otherwise known as manic depression. Both these conditions are rare before puberty. According to the mental health charity, Rethink (contact details on p. 94), symptoms of severe mental illness don't usually appear before the late teens. People with bi-polar disorder may suffer from violent mood swings which are sometimes difficult to distinguish from 'normal' teenage behaviour.

Symptoms of schizophrenia include hallucinations, hearing voices, having delusions, self-neglect and avoidance of other people, including friends and family. More information on mental illnesses can be obtained from Rethink. It points out that there is often a great deal of overlap in mental illnesses. It's not always possible even for experts to distinguish between them, or for patients and their families to obtain a clear, unchanging medical diagnosis. Their advice is *not* to wait for a diagnosis before receiving help for mental distress.

Destructive behaviour

With or without an official diagnosis of mental illness, young people under stress can behave in ways which are destructive, both of themselves and their relationships.

Symptoms of acute anxiety and distress can include:

- drinking excessively and/or using recreational drugs;
- eating disorders like anorexia and bulimia;
- self-harm – usually 'cutting' but may also include bruising, scraping, burning and other self-inflicted wounds;
- suicide or attempted suicide.

Drink and drugs

Young people have always experimented with alcohol and probably always will. We live in a heavy-drinking culture. Unlike our European neighbours, the British tend to drink in order to get drunk and young people are no exception to that rule. We hear a great deal in the media about young binge drinkers. The rise in the number of young people drinking, and the increasing amount they drink, is a cause for concern for social as well as health reasons. In the early 1990s, about 20 per cent of the 11–17-year-old age group regularly drank alcohol. More recently the figure has risen to 27 per cent, according to Alcohol Concern. The amount they drink has roughly doubled, from 5 units of alcohol a week to approximately 10. However, few studies have been done into the cause of all this drinking, and the research which does exist seems to suggest that 'binge drinking' is largely about fun and socializing. In other words, kids do it because they enjoy it and because their friends do it, rather than because they are drowning their sorrows. Having said that, there will always be a percentage of drinkers for whom alcohol is a way of blotting out their problems. Shy youngsters may find they feel more confident with a shot of 'Dutch courage' and this is where problems can begin. Alcoholics Anonymous (contact details on p. 85) can help anyone, of any age, who has a problem with drinking. Al-Anon Family Groups can also support the parents and families of problem drinkers. Frank, the national drugs helpline (contact details on p. 89) can also give information on local resources for those with a drink problem.

Most teenagers start to experiment with illegal drugs for the same reasons as they start drinking alcohol – because the drug is there, because they're curious, because their friends do, because they like the 'buzz', because they want to look cool. The effects of drugs can be unpredictable, not least because there's no quality control on dope or pills. Someone who is anxious may be made to feel much more anxious by a bad experience with a drug like LSD. Magic mushrooms, amphetamines and dance drugs like Ecstasy can also make users feel tense and panicky. According to Rethink, smoking cannabis can increase the likelihood of developing schizophrenia or schizophrenia-type symptoms in someone already at risk.

In other words, a teenager who turns to drink or drugs as a way to escape her problems is likely to find herself with *more* problems. Drug advice services are available in most areas. Call Frank, the national drugs helpline, to find out your nearest sources of help. Some are drop-in services, others are appointment-only and opening hours vary. Not all will see under-16s, with or without their parents, and rules on confidentiality vary also. Parentline Plus (contact details on p. 92) is another good source of help and advice for parents concerned about a teenager's drinking or drug habit.

Eating disorders

Many people – and not just teenagers – have a complex relationship with food. Most of us like to eat but sometimes feel guilty about eating the 'wrong' things. We worry about our weight and go on endless diets, yet the evidence is that as a nation, we are actually getting fatter. Children are sometimes rewarded for good behaviour with sweets or chocolate. Mums like to spoil their families by feeding them up.

Teenagers often experiment with new ideas about food and eating – becoming vegetarian, for example, or trying out the latest celebrity diet. This is mostly harmless and can even be beneficial, if your teenager has a craze for healthy eating! However, some youngsters – especially, but not exclusively, girls – use food and eating as a way of coping with difficult feelings and emotions as they grow up. Perhaps they are going through a hard time at school or in their relationships with friends and family. Eating disorders are not just about weight loss, they are about feelings too, and also about control.

Eating disorders are thought to affect about 60,000 people in the UK. Sometimes, the media obsession with skinny actresses, super-models and their diets is blamed for the apparent epidemic of eating disorders, but the truth seems to be somewhat more complex.

The most common eating disorders are:

- **anorexia nervosa**, where someone simply stops eating, or eats very, very little. Anorexia may begin with an ordinary attempt to slim down, but anorexics never reach their ideal weight. However skeletal they look, they still see themselves as fat. Some people with anorexia over-exercise as well. Anorexics may be preoccupied with food, talk a lot about dieting, weigh themselves frequently, and have unusual eating patterns which involve hiding food and skipping meals.
- **bulimia nervosa.** People with bulimia may eat normal or excessive amounts of food and then either make themselves sick or take large doses of laxatives in order to get rid of the calories. It's harder to recognize a bulimic as they tend to be of normal weight.
- **binge eating and compulsive over-eating.** Binge eaters and compulsive over-eaters also eat unusually large amounts of food but don't try to get rid of it by making themselves sick or taking laxatives. As a result, they often put on weight. Compulsive eaters may pick at food all the time as a way of coping with their unhappy feelings.

It goes without saying that eating disorders are bad for the health. Young people need healthy, balanced meals to develop normally. Both anorexics and bulimics can suffer from heart problems, period problems, dehydration, hypothermia, the growth of excess body hair, anaemia and gastro-intestinal problems. Untreated eating disorders can be fatal.

Many young people with eating disorders are perfectionists, who never feel their best is good enough. Taking control over what and when they eat is a way of taking control over their lives. Lack of self-esteem also contributes to their unhappiness.

Information about eating disorders and treatment for them can be obtained from the Norwich-based Eating Disorders Association (EDA) (contact details on p. 88). The EDA runs telephone helplines both for young people with eating disorders and their friends and families. There are local self-help groups, recommended books and a website. Treatment is available in hospitals, usually on an outpatient basis, though some youngsters may become in-patients for a time. Treatment is not just about helping the young person to eat normally again, but also about dealing with the issues of unhappiness, anxiety or lack of self-esteem that led to the condition developing in the first place. Help will usually be given by a team including dieticians or nutritionists, counsellors, psychiatrists and psychotherapists. In the case of young teenagers, therapy may sometimes involve the whole family.

How you can help

'Try to separate the person from the eating disorder,' says Steve Bloomfield of the EDA.

> The child you love has not changed; their illness has changed *them*. Keep the lines of communication open, even if you get abused. Your child still needs your love and support to get through this. Youngsters who have recovered from eating disorders tell us that it's vitally important they are still showed love and affection, even when their behaviour is really difficult. It gives them something to get well for.
>
> Ask for help sooner, rather than later, if you suspect your child

has an eating disorder – and be prepared for the long haul. People can and do recover but it can take five or six years and multiple admissions to hospital.

Within the family, you need to set boundaries so that everyone knows what is not acceptable behaviour – stealing food to binge on, for example. You may need to lock food away or just buy what is needed for the day. The rest of the family should be eating normal amounts of healthy food and not allow themselves to be manipulated by the person with the eating disorder. It's distressing for siblings, especially, if the sick one is always the centre of attention. Don't let yourselves be held to ransom. The EDA has a message board on its website where parents can share their tips and experiences with others.

Suicide and self-harm

In 2001, 29 under-14s and 757 young people between 15 and 24 killed themselves. Young men are especially at risk, especially those who are depressed, suffering from untreated mental health problems, or who have attempted suicide on previous occasions. The CALM helpline (contact details on p. 87) was set up specifically to help young men deal with issues of depression, stress and anxiety. Young people who kill themselves have often planned to do so for some time and many of them know someone else who has tried. Surprisingly, that puts youngsters in rural areas much higher on the 'at risk' list as, according to Samaritans, about half of them know somcone else who has attempted suicide.

A study for Samaritans of 6,000 young people in England, in 2003, found that more than one in ten (13.2 per cent) had self-harmed at some point. The most recent figures suggest that as many as 24,000 young people are admitted to hospital every year with self-inflicted injuries.

Self-harm is more common among girls and young women but psychiatrists are now beginning to realize that boys and young men are also at risk. Self-harm most commonly involves cutting, but bruising, scraping, burning or other self-inflicted damage, such as overdosing, is not uncommon either. According to mental health campaigners like SANE (contact details on p. 94), self-harm is still imperfectly understood by mental health professionals. Young people who present in A & E units having self-harmed are still being patched up and sent home without being referred for psychiatric help. Self-harmers are still sometimes seen as attention-seekers. When asked why they did it, the most usual explanations offered were 'to get relief from a terrible state of mind' or 'because I wanted to die'. For some, self-injury may be a survival strategy, a way of averting suicide when the feelings of worthlessness become too much to bear. However, people who injure themselves are at high risk of going on to commit suicide.

It is very difficult for any parent to come to terms with the idea that the child they love is so distressed that he is injuring himself or even thinking of taking his own life. Such extreme emotional distress is less common in under-12s who are less likely to self-harm or kill themselves. The Samaritans' survey found that:

- many self-harmers had friends who also injured themselves;
- they tended not to have coping strategies for dealing with problems, such as confiding their worries to friends or family. They were more likely to blame themselves, sit alone in their rooms or drink alcohol;
- they felt they had fewer people to turn to than those who did not self-harm;
- many had previously used drugs;
- they were anxious, depressed and had low self-esteem.

Samaritans is working with schools, colleges, universities and youth organizations to raise awareness of the issues around suicide and self-harm. It now refers to itself as 'the emotional support charity' and is working to improve the emotional health of children and teenagers as well as adults. It offers a 24-hour, anonymous, confidential helpline which anyone can use to talk through emotional difficulties, depression or despair. Samaritans also has an email befriending service and a presence at events popular with young people, such as the Glastonbury Festival.

There are support groups all over the country for those who self-harm, such as the National Self-Harm Network (contact details on p. 91). Mental health charities like Rethink and SANE can also offer advice and support. Rethink, for example, suggests strategies which can help self-harmers including:

- talking problems over with family, friends or other self-harmers;
- finding other ways to express feelings or release tension, such as hitting a pillow, writing, drawing or taking part in active sport;
- doing something that causes a strong feeling but is not harmful, such as crushing ice-cubes.

Britain's first large-scale enquiry into self-harm was launched in 2004 and is jointly run by the Mental Health Foundation and the Camelot Foundation. It was set up by the Government in response to rising rates of self-harm among young people and is due to report its findings in 2006.

Medication for teens with mental health problems

Young people who are diagnosed with bi-polar disorder or schizo-phrenia can be treated with drugs. According to the Royal College of Psychiatrists, medication needs to be combined with a range of therapies to help both the patient and his or her family cope with the condition. Anti-depressants or anti-psychotic drugs may be pre-scribed. There are several different ones with differing side-effects, so your child may have to try a variety of drugs before an effective treatment is found. She will probably have to take medication for some time and it's important that her treatment is reviewed regularly to make sure that it is helping and that any side-effects are manageable. If you want to know more about medication for psychiatric disorders and the options available, you can call the Psychiatric Medication Helpline for Patients and Carers (contact details on p. 93).

Other treatment for teens with mental health problems

Troubled teenagers are also likely to be treated with 'talking therapies' like psychotherapy, cognitive behaviour therapy, family therapy or supportive counselling.

As is often the case in the NHS, there may be a waiting list for treatment. According to Young Minds, some GPs prescribe medica-tion for young patients rather than letting them wait months to see a therapist. At the time of writing, just under half of young patients were seen by a specialist within four weeks and only about 10 per cent had to wait longer than six months. Young Minds is campaigning for more and better specialist mental health services for children and adolescents. At present, most NHS child psychiatrists work as part of a multi-disciplinary team which may include other specialists like child psychologists, family therapists and social workers. Most young people are treated as outpatients though there are some in-patient units for very sick and troubled youngsters.

Gavin Bayliss of Young Minds says:

We feel there should be more services for children and teenagers with mental health problems, although there are lots of people out there doing very good work within the NHS. We also believe that mental health services should be better integrated with children's services generally, so that professionals like teachers, social workers, health visitors and community workers are trained to identify low-level problems and refer young people to appropriate help. A recent initiative within the National Service Framework for children says that every area should have four 'Primary Mental Health Workers' working in community settings.

Maria's son, David, began to show symptoms of schizophrenia when he was 16.

David

When David first became ill his dad and I wondered if he had become involved with a religious cult. He began to talk a lot about saving the world and lost interest in his normal life, school and friends. He would wander off by himself at night and had to be brought home by the police several times in a very distressed state.

It seemed to take us ages to get a diagnosis though there was obviously something seriously wrong. When David began threatening suicide, I more or less demanded that he went into hospital. He had several short stays on a psychiatric ward before we managed to see a consultant who told us he had schizophrenia. We didn't know who to turn to for help, until I read about Rethink, the mental health charity, who sent us lots of useful information.

They seemed to try all sorts of drugs on David and eventually found a regime that suited him. He now has fortnightly injections, is able to live at home, and is planning to resume his studies. We know his condition can't be cured, but we hope we can all live with it.

Complementary therapies

Any complementary therapy which promotes relaxation – yoga classes, art or music therapy, acupuncture, herbal or homeopathic medicines, autogenic training – can help troubled young people as well as adults. There are few recognized clinical trials which actually prove these therapies useful, but providing any treatment is carried out by a reputable practitioner and in conjunction with conventional treatments, they can be beneficial. (For details of the organizations regulating complementary therapies, see Chapter 10.)

10
Who can help?

Having a clinging, obviously anxious child or a troubled teenager in the family can feel incredibly isolating. Help is available from the NHS and private healthcare services, but there may be a long waiting list for treatment and it can be hard to decide what kind of therapy your child needs.

What the NHS can offer

NHS child psychiatrists work in child and adolescent mental health services (CAMHS) as part of multi-disciplinary teams including other professionals such as child psychologists and social workers. Your child can be referred for help through your GP, or you could discuss your concerns with your health visitor, educational psychologist, paediatrician or social worker.

What the voluntary sector can offer

Because of the isolation experienced by those with mental health problems and their parents and carers, there is an enormous amount of help available from voluntary organizations. That doesn't just mean those with a special interest in mental and emotional health like Young Minds and Samaritans, but also those which help people to cope with situations which produce anxiety, from illness and bereavement to bullying and divorce. There are organizations designed to support parents and websites for troubled teenagers. Most offer a combination of practical advice from experts – or information about where such advice can be found – and 'self-help', often shared with others who have come through the same problems themselves. Anxiety may be isolating, but the truth is that you and your anxious child are not alone.

The following organizations may be able to help you.

Action for Sick Children
3 Abbey Business Centre
Keats Lane
Earl Shilton
Leics. LE9 7DQ
Tel: 0800 074 4519
Website: www.actionforsickchildren.org

Campaigns for better healthcare for children and teenagers, including issues like hospital car-parking for parents. Produces booklets and leaflets for sick and hospitalized children and their parents.

Al-Anon Family Groups UK and Eire
61 Great Dover Street
London SE1 4YF
Tel: 020 7403 0888
Website: www.al-anonuk.org.uk

Offers support to those concerned about a family member's drinking.

Alcoholics Anonymous
PO Box 1
Stonebow House
Stonebow
York YO1 7NJ
Tel: 0845 769 7555
Website: www.alcoholics-anonymous.org.uk

Helps people of any age with a drink problem.

Blue Cross Pet Bereavement
Shilton Road
Burford
Oxfordshire OX18 4PF
Helpline: 0800 096 6606
Website: www.bluecross.org.uk

British Acupuncture Council
63 Jeddo Road
London W12 9HQ

Tel: 020 8735 0400
Website: www.acupuncture.org.uk

Can put you in touch with an accredited acupuncturist in your area.

British Association of Art Therapists
24–27 White Lion Street
London N1 9PD
Tel: 020 7686 4216
Website: www.baat.org

Can give information about art therapy in your area.

British Homeopathic Association
Hahnemann House
29 Park Street West
Luton
Bedfordshire LU1 3BE
Tel: 0870 444 3950
Website: www.trusthomeopathy.org

Can give details of registered practitioners in your area.

British Red Cross
44 Moorfields
London EC2Y 9AL
Tel: 0870 170 7000
Website: www.redcross.org.uk/babysitting

Gives details of babysitting courses.

British Society for Music Therapy
61 Church Hill Road
East Barnet
Hertfordshire EN4 8SY
Tel: 020 8441 6226
Website: www.bsmt.org

Can put you in touch with a music therapist in your area.

British Wheel of Yoga
25 Jermyn Street
Sleaford
Lincolnshire NG34 7RU
Tel: 01529 306851
Website: www.bwy.org.uk

Can give information about local yoga teachers and classes.

Brook Advisory Centres
421 Highgate Studios
53–79 Highgate Road
London NW5 1TL
Tel: 0800 0185 023
Website: www.brook.org.uk

Free and confidential advice for young people on contraception and sexual health.

CALM Helpline
0800 58 58 58
Website: www.thecalmzone.net

Open from 5 p.m. to 3 a.m. every day, this is a helpline for troubled and worried young people, especially young men.

CancerBACUP
3 Bath Place
Rivington Street
London EC2A 3JR
Helpline: 0808 800 1234
Website: www.cancerbacup.org

Offers support and information about cancer including useful booklets such as *What Do I Tell the Children?*.

ChildLine
45 Folgate Street
London E1 6GL
Tel: 0800 1111
Website: www.childline.org.uk

Offers help to children in trouble or danger. Of the calls to their helpline every year, 31,000 concern bullying.

Children's Legal Centre
University of Essex
Wivenhoe Park
Colchester
Essex CO4 3SQ
Tel: 01206 872 466
Education Law Advice Line: 0845 456 6811
Website: www.childrenslegalcentre.com

Information and advice on parental responsibility and children's rights.

Cruse Bereavement Care
Cruse House
126 Sheen Road
Richmond
Surrey TW9 1UR
Helpline: 0870 167 1677 (adults); 0808 808 1677 (young people)
Website: www.crusebereavementcare.org.uk; www.rd4u.org.uk
(young people)

Offers help and support to anyone who has been bereaved, including booklets for children and teenagers.

Dept of Education & Skills
Caxton House
Tothill Street
London SW1H 9NA
Tel: 0845 602 2260
Website: www.dfes.gov.uk/bullying

Has produced an anti-bullying pack available to parents, teachers and young people.

Eating Disorders Association
First Floor, Wensum House
103 Prince of Wales Road
Norwich NR1 1DW
Tel: 0845 634 7650 (for under-18s)
    0845 634 1414 (for over-18s)
Website: www.edauk.com

Supports those with eating disorders and their families.

Education Otherwise
PO Box 7420
London N9 9SG
Tel: 0870 730 0074
Website: www.education-otherwise.org

Information and support for parents who want to educate their children at home.

Family Welfare Association
501–505 Kingsland Road
London E8 4AU
Tel: 020 7254 6251
Website: www.fwa.org.uk

Provides both practical and emotional support for vulnerable and/or disadvantaged children and their parents.

FPA
2–12 Pentonville Road
London N1 9FP
Helpline: 0845 310 1334
Website: www.fpa.org.uk

Has information about all aspects of sexual health, including contraception, with special leaflets for teenagers, both boys and girls.

Frank, the national drugs helpline
Helpline: 0800 77 66 00
Website: www.talktofrank.com

Free, confidential advice and information on drugs, available 24 hours a day.

Hyperactive Children's Support Group
71 Whyke Lane
Chichester
West Sussex PO19 7PD
Tel: 01243 539966
Website: www.hacsg.org.uk

Offers help to parents of children with attention deficit hyperactivity disorder and similar conditions.

Kidscape
2 Grosvenor Gardens
London SW1W 0DH
Helpline: 08451 205 204
Website: www.kidscape.org.uk

Campaigns on all aspects of children's safety, including information about bullying and all kinds of child abuse.

Learndirect
Tel: 0800 100 900
Website: www.learndirect.co.uk

Information about college courses of all kinds, plus careers guidance.

The Multiple Sclerosis Society
Information Team
MS National Centre
372 Edgware Road
Staples Corner
London NW2 6ND
Helpline: 0808 800 8000
Website: www.mssociety.org.uk

Nacro
169 Clapham Road
London SW9 0PU
Tel: 020 7582 6500
Website: www.nacro.org.uk

Crime reduction charity providing activities for young people excluded from school or at risk of drifting into crime.

National Childminding Association
8 Masons Hill
Bromley

Kent BR2 9EY
Tel: 0800 169 4486
Website: www.ncma.org.uk

Has information about helping your child settle in with a child-minder.

National Family Mediation
Tel: 01392 668090
Website: www.nfm.u-net.com

Has a network of 57 mediation services around the country. Trained mediators can help separating and divorcing couples to make the best arrangements for their children.

National Institute of Medical Herbalists
Elm House
54 Mary Arches Street
Exeter
Devon EX4 3BA
Tel: 01392 426022
Website: www.nimh.org.uk

Can refer you to a qualified medical herbalist in your area.

National Pyramid Trust
84 Uxbridge Road
London W13 8RA
Tel: 020 8579 5108
Website: www.nptrust.org.uk

Runs 'Pyramid Clubs', through schools, for children between 7 and 11 who seem withdrawn, isolated or have emotional problems, aiming to raise their self-esteem. The trust also runs parents' support groups.

National Self-Harm Network
PO Box 7264
Nottingham NG1 6WJ
Website: www.nshn.co.uk

The network was set up to benefit self-harm survivors and their families.

NCH
85 Highbury Park
London N5 1UD
Tel: 020 7704 7000
Website: www.nch.org.uk

No Panic
93 Brands Farm Way
Telford
Shropshire TF3 2JQ
Tel: 0808 808 0545
Website: www.nopanic.org.uk

Help for anyone suffering from phobias and panic attacks.

NSPCC
Weston House
42 Curtain Road
London EC2A 3NH
24-hour Child Protection Helpline: 0808 800 5000
Website: www.nspcc.org.uk

Campaigns against all forms of child abuse. Has a useful range of leaflets for parents and young people.

Parentline Plus
520 Highgate Studios
53–79 Highgate Road
London NW5 1TL
Helpline: 0808 800 2222
Website: www.parentlineplus.org.uk

Offers help with all aspects of parenting, including divorce and separation, bullying, discipline, step-parenting, plus forums where parents can contact others in the same situation.

Positive Parenting
2a South Street
Gosport PO12 1ES
Tel: 023 9252 8787
Website: www.parenting.org.uk

Produces helpful leaflets for parents and professionals and also runs parenting workshops.

Princess Royal Trust for Carers
142 Minories
London EC3N 1LB
Tel: 020 7480 7788
Website: www.youngcarers.net

Has around 70 projects around the country for 'young carers' who care for sick or disabled relatives.

Psychiatric Medication Helpline for Patients and Carers
Maudsley Hospital
Denmark Hill
London SE5 8AZ
020 7919 2999

For expert information about treatment options for those with mental health problems.

Relate
Tel: 01788 573241
Website: www.relate.org

Help for anyone with relationship problems, including separation and divorce.

Re-Solv
30a High Street
Stone
Staffordshire ST15 8AW
Helpline: 0808 800 2345
Website: www.re-solv.org (for parents)
Website: www.sniffing.org.uk (for young people)

Help for parents and children concerned about solvent abuse.

Rethink
30 Tabernacle Street
London EC2A 4DD
Tel: 0845 456 0455
Website: www.rethink.org

Campaigns on behalf of those with severe mental illness and has many useful booklets about mental disorders such as schizophrenia.

RoSPA Information Centre
353 Bristol Road
Edgbaston
Birmingham B5 7ST
Tel: 0121 248 2000
Website: www.rospa.com

As well as information about accident prevention, it has a leaflet, *The RoSPA Guide to Good Practice in Babysitting*, which is free in return for a large sae.

Samaritans
The Upper Mill
Kingston Road
Ewell
Surrey KT17 2AF
Tel: 08457 90 90 90
Website: www.samaritans.org

Offers 24-hour, totally confidential support and a listening ear to anyone in emotional distress.

SANE
1st Floor, Cityside House
40 Adler Street
London E1 1EE
Tel: 0845 767 8000
Website: www.sane.org.uk

Campaigns to improve the quality of life for those affected by mental illness, including families.

Suzy Lamplugh Trust
PO Box 17818
London SW14 8WW
Tel: 020 8876 0305
Website: www.suzylamplugh.org

Charity which gives advice on personal safety. Not specifically for young people, but many of their leaflets give useful advice for teenagers.

Teenage Cancer Trust
38 Warren Street
London W1T 6AE
Tel: 020 7387 1000
Website: www.teenagecancertrust.org

Builds dedicated units for teenage cancer patients in hospitals and also runs Education and Awareness teams and support for families.

Victim Support
Cranmer House
39 Brixton Road
London SW9 6DZ
Tel: 0845 30 30 900
Website: www.victimsupport.org

Trained volunteers can offer practical help and support to victims of crime, including support in going to court.

Winston's Wish
Clara Burgess Centre
Bayshill Road
Cheltenham
Gloucestershire GL50 3AW
Tel: 0845 20 30 40 5
Website: www.winstonswish.org.uk

Supports bereaved children and young people.

YoungMinds
48–50 St John Street

London EC1M 4DG
Tel: 020 7336 8445
Parents Information Service: 0800 018 2138
Website: www.youngminds.org.uk

Information and advice about all forms of mental and emotional distress in young people.

Youth Access
1–2 Taylors Yard
67 Alderbrook Road
London SW12 8AD
Tel: 020 8772 9900
Website: www.youthaccess.org.uk

Has a directory of young people's advice services and can refer the 11–25 age group to support services all over Britain.

Websites
There are also lots of independent websites to help parents and young people cope with anxiety and other emotional difficulties as well as those listed above. You could take a look at:

www.childanxiety.net

www.parentscentre.gov.uk

www.raisingkids.co.uk

www.safekids.com

Teenagers might like to check out:

www.itsnotyourfault.co.uk

www.lifebytes.gov.uk

www.teenagehealthfreak.org

www.there4me.com

www.thesite.org

Helpful books

Barrell, Sarah, *Brothers and Sisters*. Oxford, 2004 (available from: PO Box 95, Witney, Oxon OX29 4WJ).

Furedi, Frank, *Paranoid Parenting*. Allen Lane/The Penguin Press, London, 2001.

Index